HOMŒOPATHIC TREATMENT

OF

EPIDEMIC CHOLERA,

By B. F. JOSLIN, M.D., L.L.D.,

FELLOW OF THE ALBANY MEDICAL COLLEGE; FELLOW AND CORRESPONDING MEMBER OF THE HOMŒOPATHIC MEDICAL COLLEGE OF PENNSYLVANIA, &c., &c.

THIRD EDITION, WITH ADDITIONS.

NEW-YORK:

PUBLISHED BY WILLIAM RADDE, No. 322 BROADWAY.

PHILADELPHIA: RADEMACHER & SHEEK.—BOSTON: OTIS CLAPP.—LONDON: J. EPPS, 112 GREAT RUSSELL-ST., BLOOMSBURY.—MANCHESTER: HENRY TURNER, 41 PICCADILLY.

1854.

HENRY LUDWIG, Printer, 45 Vesey-street.

CONTENTS.

PREFACE AND INTRODUCTION.

The favorable reception which the former editions of this book have met with, has encouraged the author in the labor of improving it, by such modifications and additions as were suggested by much experience in the epidemic of 1849. A great amount of practical matter has been added, including a chapter of illustrative cases, in 1849 and subsequent years, to the present month.

The book has been used as a guide in the treatment of cholera, not only by the profession, but by many intelligent laymen. In this rapid disease, for which our system affords the only effectual remedies, many families in localities where no homœopathic physician can be soon procured, will find it necessary at last to commence the treatment; and some members of the profession who had been previously allopathic will be induced to prescribe homœopathically for cholera. In consideration of the wants of these two classes, the more important rules of treatment are given in a more particular and elementary form, than would be necessary for an experienced homœopathic practitioner. The plain rules for prevention, preliminary treatment and nursing, may either be consulted directly by families, or employed by their physician as a safe and convenient basis for his instructions.

The plan offers the advantage of a threefold arrangement of the principal medicines; viz., with reference, 1st, to the varieties of cholera; 2d, to its stages; and 3d, to its symptoms as arranged in repertories. These last will give the work a permanent value, in treating the more frequent complaints of summer. The author has aimed to prepare for the use of practitioners a portable treatise, so full and systematic as to enable them to find with facility the remedy for every curable case of this disease.

When we fail in our attempts at homœopathic treatment, in any malady which is curable in the present state of the Materia Medica, the fault is not in the law, but in its administration. It is unjust in any one, to impute to Homœopathy the disastrous consequences of his own ignorance, indolence or haste, and unwise to attempt by allopathic patches to strengthen his practice already sufficiently spurious, and consequently feeble. Such expedients emasculate his Homœopathy. None will learn to swim who depend upon bladders under the arms. Eclecticism will be less resorted to, in proportion as the character of the profession shall become more elevated in intellect, industry and attainments, and physicians shall not consider a minute study of the case and of the Materia Medica too onerous, when human life depends on the correctness of the prescription. With Hahnemann's eulogium of the profession, he has connected a requirement and an injunction. "To the physician, whose province it is to vanquish the disease that brings its victim to the very borders of corporeal dissolution, and to produce as it were a second creation of life—a greater work than almost all the other much-vaunted performances of mankind—to him Nature in all her wide expanse, with all her sources and productions must lie open. Let all hold aloof from this most pious, this noblest of all secular professions, who are deficient in mind, in patient thought, in the requisite knowledge, or in tender philanthropy and a sense of duty." However great may be the general attainments of a physician, there is one kind of knowledge indispensable, that of the Materia Medica: and as none but a charlatan affects to be able to retain an adequate amount of it in his mind, the best physicians study it at the bed-side of the sick, and partly in a repertory, a Materia Medica in which the symptoms have an orderly arrangement, for convenience of reference and greater certainty in the selection of the *best* remedy.

The Homœopathic Materia Medica is the true test of the correctness of conclusions drawn from Clinical experience; indeed, it was originally the only guide to that practice which was attended with such splendid results in 1832. It was Hahnemann's confidence in this, and in his law of cure, that enabled him to publish the plan on which this fearful malady was successfully combated. With his usual sagacity, he pointed out the true prophylactics, and all the most important curatives, when this pestilence had not fallen under his own observation. Having discovered and demonstrated a universal, unerring, and everlasting law in medicine, he was prepared to encounter the strangest forms of disease as though they were familiar. The law is *similia similibus curantur*, like are cured by like; or (to expand this brief and elliptical aphorism) diseases are cured by medicines which tend to excite affections similar to the diseases themselves. From the Greek ὁμοιον πάθος (homoion pathos, affectus similis, the Latin term Homœopathia, and the English Homœopathy, are derived.

We frequently hear persons who have no experience in Homœopathy, or who at most have seen its effect in Chronic cases, saying, I would not dare to trust it if I were very sick, with a dangerous and rapid disease. I should want something that would act powerfully and quickly. A potentized medicine selected in accordance with the Homœopathic law, is that very thing. Thousands of physicians know it to be such; and that in their own former Allœopathic practice, and in that of their brethren of the old school, no violent and rapid diseases have been cured as surely and promptly as they now cure them by the homœopathic method. Large doses are not required to cure any disease whatever. Attenuation, whilst it weakens and ultimately nullifies poisons, as such, is in almost every substance essential to the full development of medicinal power; and, in some substances, no medicinal power whatever is manifested until the substance is rendered extremely dilute. This book will contain abundant experimental evidence of the efficacy of attenuated medicines in the treatment of Cholera. The great success of European physicians in the treatment of the Asiatic Cholera of 1832, and of many American physicians in 1849, was due to the use of attenuated medicines, as well as to the law of similitude which regulated their administration. If the author were charged with the duty of testing the relative merits of the homœopathic and allopathic laws of cure before an impartial and intelligent tribunal of either school, and if his life depended upon obtaining a verdict in favor of Homœopathy, he would not only select violent and rapid diseases, in preference to such as are mild and chronic, but would administer attenuated medicines, in small doses.

As the potencies and doses recommended by Dr. QUIN of London, and on his authority in the former editions of this book, have with all who employed them in 1849, well sustained the reputation gained in 1832, they have not been changed in the present edition.* In the present state of homœopathic science they may be properly denominated the medium dilutions. Those who prefer lower or higher ones, will find no difficulty in using this book as a guide in the selection and administration of the remedies. The same number of globules and the same intervals between the doses, will be appropriate.

New-York, July, 1854.

---

* Other acknowledgements of some of the advantages, which this book has derived from the excellent French treatise, of this distinguished and venerated pioneer of sound Homœopathy in England, are given on pages, 71, 121, 122, 123 and 170.

LIST OF THE CHOLERA MEDICINES,

WITH THE PROPER ATTENUATIONS.

Names.			*Abbreviations.*
Aconitum, 24th attenuation ;		"	Acon. ^{24}
Arsenicum, 30th ;	"	"	*Ars.* ^{30}
Belladonna, 30th ;	"	"	Bell. ^{30}
Camphora, Tinct. & 3d,	"	"	Camph ^{0} & ^{3}
Cantharis, 30th ;	"	"	Canth. ^{30}
Carbo-vegetabilis, 30th ;	"	"	*Carb-v.* ^{30}
Chamomilla, 30th ;	"	"	Cham. ^{30}
Cicuta, 30th ;	"	"	Cic. ^{30}
Cinchona, 12th ;	"	"	Cin. ^{12}
CUPRUM, 30th ;	"	"	CUPR. ^{30}
Acidum-hydrocianicum, 30th ;		"	Hydrocy. ^{30}
Ipecacuanha, 3d,	"	"	*Ipec.* ^{3}
Jatropha, 12th ;	"	"	*Jat.* ^{12}
Mercurius-vivus, 12th ;	"	"	Merc. ^{12}
Natrum-muriaticum, 12th ;	"	"	Natr-m. ^{12}
Nux-vomica, 30th ;	"	"	Nux, ^{30}
PHOSPHORUS, 30th ;	"	"	PHOS. ^{30}
PHOSPHORI-ACIDUM, 3d, & 30th ;		"	PHOS.-AC. ^{3} & ^{30}
Rhus-radicans, 30th ;	"	"	R.-rad. ^{30}
Secale-cornutum, 12th ;	"	"	*Sec.* ^{12}
Stramonium, 12th ;	"	"	Stram. ^{12}
Sulphur, 30th ;	"	"	Sulph. ^{30}
Tartarus-emeticus, 12th ;	"	"	Tart. ^{12}
VERATRUM, 12th & 30th		"	VERAT. ^{12} & ^{30}

* The distinctions of type refer to the more or less frequent demand for these medicines in the disease proper. This elevated location of the figures in the last column, promotes brevity and prevents ambiguity, where other figures or words follow. It is also appropriate, as the number is the mathematical exponent of that power of 100 which expresses the degree of dilution, and of that power of 1/100, which expresses the quantity of the medicinal basis contained in the preparation.

CHAPTER I.

NATURE AND PATHOLOGY OF CHOLERA,

WITH REFERENCE TO THE DARK COLOR OF THE BLOOD AND THE DEFICIENCY OF ANIMAL HEAT.

CHARACTERISTICS.

THE disease which is now generally known by the name of Cholera, or The Cholera, and which has been denominated Epidemic, Asiatic, Spasmodic and Pestilential Cholera, and Cholera Asphyctica or Asphyxia, agrees in but few particulars with the ordinary Sporadic or Bilious Cholera, known by the name of Cholera Morbus. It usually differs from the latter in the whitish appearance of the alvine evacuations; in the absence of bile in them and in the matters vomited; and the suppression of other secretions, especially that of the urine; in the greater liability to cramps and other spasms; in the coldness of the body, including surface, tongue, breath, &c.; in the livid color of the skin; in the early cessation of the pulse; and in the great rapidity and fatality of the disease.

Dissections reveal but few and slight traces of inflammation or other morbid changes in the solid constituents of the bodies of persons who have died of this disease—none that are constant, and in many cases none at all.

Hence the disease is calculated to confute the theory and paralyze the exertions of the anatomical sect. It is found no less puzzling and intractable by the chemical and mechanical sects; although they have given some attention to the blood, the part in which the most important morbid alterations are found. The chemical Allopathists have endeavored to supply the deficiency of its salts by artificially introducing them, either by the mouth or the veins; whilst the mechanical Allopathists, supposing that the thickening of the blood was merely a consequence of the discharge of its watery parts into the intestines, strive to arrest this discharge by opiates and astringents. The most pure and perfect specimen of this practice, is a plan proposed by an Allopathic medical professor: viz., to cork up the anus.

The hints I have to offer on the pathology of this disease may be of some use, if they serve no other purpose but to dissuade from such mechanical views, and teach that no reliance can be placed on any treatment but that which is specific in its nature and symptomatic in its rule, and which, under the guidance of an unerring law, strikes at the secret springs of morbid action. A consideration of the true source of animal heat will show the futility of all attempts to restore it by hot baths or hot drinks, whilst the vital and chemical processes on which it depends continue to be interrupted—to say nothing of the delusive analogy between actual warmth and that sensation of warmth which is produced by stimulants, and which has led some to attach some importance to these in Cholera.

Another object will be, to point out such relations between certain pathological and ætiological facts, as will afford some clue to the apparently anomalous character of the predisposing causes, to impress the importance of certain precautionary measures relating to diet and regimen, and afford aid in prognosticating the progress of the epidemic.

One of the most remarkable features of *Cholera* in an advanced stage, and of the more perfect types of the disease almost immediately after its onset, is the rapid failure of *animal heat.* The temperature of the whole body is greatly reduced, and some parts acquire a marbly coldness long before death. The coldness of the skin, tongue, breath, &c., I have frequently observed, and others have a thousand times described. These phenomena must be attributed to some impression which the poison—probably introduced through the lungs into the blood—has made upon the nervous system; an impression which interferes with the introduction of oxygen into the blood, or with its chemical action on the carbon and hydrogen.

PHYSIOLOGY OF RESPIRATION.

With respect to *animal heat in general*, the results of Mr. Brodie's experiments were, for a while, thought by many to be fatal to every modification of the chemical theory, from those of Black and Lavoisier to that of Crawford. But the later and more careful experiments and more correct reasonings of Drs. Philip, Legallois, Edwards, and Liebig, have tended to restore the chemical theory, so far at least as it respects the general doctrine of the dependence of calorification on the absorption of oxygen and the production of carbonic acid. But although respiration must be considered essential to animal heat, some physiologists are still disposed to attribute calorification, in part, to the direct actions of the nervous and circulatory systems. The influence of these, however, appears to be indirect. The contact and combination of the oxygen with the blood, is promoted by innervation and circulation, whilst the latter diffuses through the system that caloric, which by the union of oxygen with carbon and hydrogen, is evolved on the same principle as in combustion.

Without dwelling upon the analogy between respiration and combustion, or upon the influence of hydrogen, it will be sufficient barely to allude to a few of the numerous experiments and observations, which prove a necessary *relation* between the amount of *carbonic acid* produced during respiration and that of *caloric* evolved in the system. For example, Legallois effected a diminution in both, by placing an animal in such a position as constrained its respiration. Edwards ascertained that both were affected in a corresponding manner by the influence of the seasons: for in summer, less carbonic acid was formed, and likewise less heat was evolved. The latter fact was not a mere inference from the former, but was established by exposing the same kind of animal to the same freezing mixture in winter and in summer, and finding that in the latter season, the reduction of its temperature was, in a given time, six or eight times as great as in winter.

The *final cause* of this correspondence between the oxygen consumed and the temperature of the surrounding medium, is as obvious as it is interesting. This is a beneficent provision, by which, as well as by a variable cutaneous and pulmonary transpiration, the Author of nature has, in some degree, defended man and the inferior animals against the vicissitudes of the seasons. But neither our limits nor the nature of our subject will allow us to dwell upon this interesting topic.

That correspondence between the degrees of aëration and those of animal heat, which has been already alluded to, *extends to the whole animal kingdom.* It will be found to exist, whether we compare the warm-blooded animals with those called cold-blooded, or the different species of either of these grand divisions with each other. The respiration of the lower orders of animals is, however, so imperfect, and their temperature is, consequently, so little elevated above that of the media in which they reside, that the evidence of the extension of the above law to them was at one time merely analogical. But discoveries in electro-magnetism have suggested an extremely delicate thermometer, by means of which, the relation' that in the higher classes of animals, is known to exist between animal heat and aëration, is proved to hold even among different species of insects as compared with each other; those which produce more carbonic acid, possess a more elevated temperature. This may therefore be regarded as a universal law.

There is no difficulty in understanding why the skin should have a dark color, whenever the deficiency of animal heat in the body, and of the oxygen used and the carbonic acid formed during respiration, evince an accumulation of carbon in the blood.

APPLICATION TO THE PATHOLOGY OF CHOLERA.

That *a dark color of the blood is one of the characteristics of Cholera*, is well known. To this color of the blood we are to attribute the livid color of the surface of the body—a color which is not, however, identical with that of the blood, but depends partly upon the color of the medium through which the blood is seen.

In this disease, there is frequently no sensible difference between the color of the venous and that of the arterial blood. Many physicians have compared the blood to tar or treacle. The blood drawn from a patient was found by Dr. Reid Clanny to be as black as tar, and to contain more than twice as much carbon as healthy blood. It was tasteless, and contained no carbonic acid or gas of any kind. The want of taste cannot be wholly referred to the elimination of salts, but affords evidence of a defect in the respiratory function; for the stronger taste is one of the properties acquired by this liquid in traversing the lungs; and as superior sapidity distinguishes arterial from venous blood, we might naturally expect it to distinguish venous blood from supervenous.

Whether the carbon which he obtained by his ultimate analysis, previously existed in a free state, as he, in my opinion, too hastily concluded, is of little consequence. None of those who have objected to his views, have produced any ultimate analysis which militates against his conclusion, that there is a great excess of carbon, compared with that which exists in normal blood. In the controversy which has been carried on by Dr. Clanny and others, the object has been, either to prove or disprove the existence of carbon in the blood in a *free* state, and the excess of *uncombined* carbon in cholera blood. The decision of this point is probably of little importance in the pathology of Cholera; at any rate, it does not, in the least, affect the question which I am considering. The manner in which the elements of that part of the coloring matter which contains carbon, are arranged, whether in binary, ternary or quaternary combination, has never been determined; but Brande, Engelhart and Michaelis have shown that the coloring matter of the blood consists of an animal matter, associated with a minute quantity of iron and some earthy salts; and this animal matter, of which the coloring matter appears chiefly to consist, was found by Michaelis to contain more than fifty-three per cent. of carbon. Now in what degree the carbon of the coloring matter may vary in different kinds of blood, I find no satisfactory data for determining. The furnishing of these is, perhaps, a service which pathology has yet to expect from chemistry. But even conceding, that a given quantity of the coloring matter of cholera blood, contains only the same amount of carbon as the same quantity of the coloring matter of normal blood, (and no one has pretended that it contains less,) it can, I think, be shown, that the whole amount of carbon in the coloring matter of the former, far exceeds the whole amount in the coloring matter of the latter. For according to the researches of Dr. Thompson, professor of Chemistry in Glasgow, the coloring matter of cholera blood, as deduced from the mean of his results, is "little short of *four times* the quantity of coloring matter of healthy blood." Dr. Clanny's *proximate* analysis afforded nearly the same result. This may be reconciled with the result of his *destructive* distillation in another instance, in which he obtained only about twice as much carbon from cholera blood as from healthy blood, by considering that both fibrine and albumen contain rather more than fifty per cent. of carbon, and that the great increase of coloring matter, is partly compensated by the diminution of the sum of these other carbonaceous principles. That this will explain the apparent discrepancy, might be shown by the numerical results. But that the change in the absolute amount of fibrine is small, compared with that of the coloring matter, is evident from Dr. Thompson's testimony, that the fibrine and coloring matter of healthy blood added together, amount to less than one-half the coloring matter in cholera blood. Notwithstanding all that has been said by the opponents of hyperanthraxis, I am unable to discern, why the quantities of carbon obtained from two portions of blood, submitted under the same circumstances, to destructive distillation in a close vessel, may not correctly show the relative proportions that actually existed in them. The only sound objection refers to the *state* in which the carbon existed.

Now, that this vast accumulation of carbon in the blood of a cholera patient is absolute, and not merely a relative increase, resulting from incrassation, in consequence of the removal of its aqueous portion, by profuse evacuations or any other cause, we may readily convince ourselves from a comparison of the numerical results in Dr. Thompson's table, by which it will be found, that the proportional diminution of water in cholera blood is very small, compared either

2*

with the proportional increase of coloring matter as shown by his experiments, or of carbon as shown by Dr. Clanny's. How then can it be true, that the addition of the dejections to the blood would restore it to its normal condition? Are not even Dr. O'Shaugnessy's results with respect to the albumen, opposed to the above conclusion which has been drawn from his analysis? The *history* of this epidemic is opposed to it. It has been long since and repeatedly observed, by those who have been familiar with the disease in its most malignant and perfect form, that the most rapid and intractable cases were generally attended with slight, if any, alvine evacuations. Not to cite other authorities, Mr. Orton, at Bombay, and other surgeons in that vicinity, stated that in many cases there was no purging, in some no vomiting, and in others neither, and that these were by far the most dangerous cases, and that the patients died under them, often in an hour or two; and that, without spasms and with scarcely any vomiting or purging, all the secretions appeared to be in many cases entirely suspended.* Conceding the possibility, that in some cases, the contents of the alimentary canal may not have been examined, still, from what we know of its dimensions, and from the effects of equivalent evacuations in other diseases, a theory which can be defended only by a supposed accumulation in such cases, must be considered untenable. Has it

*Good's Study of Med. I. 178.

not been chiefly in those places which have been but slightly visited, that we find pathologists disposed to found a theory on profuse evacuations? Under such circumstances, these may perhaps merit all the attention which has been bestowed upon them; although the most fatal alterations of the blood, and the suppression of urine and other secretions, must often, if not always, depend upon another cause.*

It is hardly necessary to remark, that the presence of an immense excess of carbon in the blood, manifests a defect in the decarbonizing process of the system. It may be less obvious, though hardly less certain, that the observed *absence of carbonic acid* in the blood, in this disease, depends upon a similar cause. A considerable quantity of this gas exists in healthy blood; and it might be asked, why the same cause, from which, in this disease, the blood retains its carbon, does not also make it retain the carbonic acid. I answer, it is because the carbonic acid elimi-

* There is little doubt that the secretion of urine may be both increased and diminished, by some agencies which have no direct influence on the action of the kidneys, or the quantity of serum in the blood. Even Dr. Cullen acknowledged his suspicion of this, opposed as it was to his favorite theory. His modesty and candor are worthy of the imitation of those who are ambitious of framing *complete* theories in medicine. He says, that "besides the increased quantity of water in the mass of the blood, or a stimulus particularly applied to the kidneys, there may be a medicine which, by a general operation on the system, may promote the secretion of urine.—My candor obliges me to mention this; but I do not find myself at present in a condition to prosecute the inquiry.—Materia Med. vol. p. 556.

nated during respiration, derives its oxygen from the inspired air; and when little or no oxygen is absorbed, we should expect little or no carbonic acid to be formed. From the absence or deficiency of carbonic acid, I should infer, that in this disease, there exists *more difficulty in obtaining the advantages of inspiration* than those of expiration—in forming carbonic acid than in eliminating it.

In the phenomena presented after death, there are many striking coincidences between Cholera and asphyxia from other causes; the same fluidity of the blood, for hours after death, the same tendency of the body after death to an increase of warmth and diminution of lividity, as in cases where the respiration is suspended by hanging or drowning, or not established by a closure of the foramen ovale. I have known these phenomena to be presented after death in the case of a premature child, which was born at the end of the 7th month, and lived till the fourth day after its birth; and I have observed some of them in cases of death by hanging and drowning, and I believe them to be characteristic of asphyxia. They frequently inspire the friends of the deceased with the vain hope of effecting a resuscitation.

The following case will illustrate some of the foregoing remarks, as well as the effect produced on the blood by certain salts, which, since the experiments of Dr. Stevens, have been supposed to perform an important part in the function of respiration. A son of Mr. V. V., ætat. eighteen months, had fallen into a cistern of water, and lain, as was supposed, a quarter of an hour or more, and had been taken out about half an hour before my arrival. We attempted to re-establish respiration, by inflating the lungs, not only by the mouth, but by a pair of bellows fitted to a flexible tube which was introduced into the trachea. Other means were used, but to no effect. About two hours after the death of the child, the jugular vein was opened. A dark-colored blood ran freely. Three or four ounces were taken. Its coagulability was so slight, that it required a plaster to arrest it. As the plasticity or coagulability of arterial blood as compared with venous, is a property acquired by respiration, it might be expected, that the supervenous blood of Cholera and other species of asphyxia, would be more deficient in this property than ordinary venous blood. And such is the fact. In the above case, it coagulated very slowly and imperfectly after its removal from the vein, resembling, in this respect, the blood drawn during life from Cholera patients. After half an hour had elapsed, about one-third of it had not coagulated, although the temperature of the air was about 70°. The upper part, which had been exposed to the air, was coagulated to a certain depth, and its color at the surface had become rather brighter. On inclining the vessel, the dark, thick and uncoagulated fluid broke through the coagulated crust, and flowed sluggishly across it, presenting an appearance somewhat similar to that of Cholera blood, which from its consistence and blackness, has so often been compared to molasses and tar. The parts of the coagulum below the surface were also dark-colored. It appeared evident, that air favored coagulation, and was more essential to the production of the florid color, but did not appear to effect the latter as readily and perfectly as in the case of normal or healthy blood. Muriate of soda was then added to one portion, and carbonate of soda to another. The latter had a marked effect, rendering it florid. This experiment, and others made on normal venous blood, have convinced me that it is unphilosophical to infer from the effect of salts in reddening cholera blood, that the asphyxia which produces its dark color depends on the deficiency of saline ingredients in the blood, even though such deficiency should by analysis be shown to exist; for in the case above mentioned, and in others alluded to, a similar change of color was produced by the salts, although there was no reason to suspect any greater deficiency of saline ingredients than ordinarily exists in venous blood. The circumstance that the color of the blood was less influenced by exposure to air than ordinary venous blood, shows that a defect in this property is not peculiar to Cholera, nor to disease of any kind, properly so called, but appears to be characteristic of asphyxia in general, whether induced by disease or suddenly caused by interrupting the respiration of an individual previously in health, when there have been no intestinal discharges to drain the salts from the system.

I consider the defect in coagulability as also common to all those cases where a want of due oxygenation is the sole or chief cause of death. Excessive exercise and violent mental emotions, when they occur suddenly, are said to produce this state of the blood; and it appears to me an interesting fact, that these are also among the causes which tend to prevent its oxygenation. Another correspondence not less curious is, that in the fœtus, whose respiration has never been established, the venous and arterial blood, like that of the victims of Cholera, is nearly identical; the blood is not coagulable, has an unctuous feel, and does not take the vermilion color on exposure to the air; and according to Fourcroy, it has its coloring matter darker and more abundant, and contains no fibrine. It therefore remarkably resembles Cholera blood. Would it not seem, from these facts and considerations, that the coagulation of the fibrine, and even its existence as such, are more dependent on respiration than has been hitherto suspected; and that the deficiency of this principle, as well as the existence of most of the other peculiarities which distinguish cholera blood from normal blood, result chiefly from its defective aëration, and are what might be expected in asphyxia from any other cause? Dr. Good admits the want of coagulability of the blood in cases of electrical, and Broussais in cases of gaseous asphyxia. Combining these two authorities, relating respectively to asphyxia caused by lightning and that caused by the irrespirable and deleterious gases, with my own observations on other varieties of asphyxia, I am led to infer the generality of the above law. That the tarry appearance of cholera blood results from want of aëration, is also confirmed by the fact, that the same appearance may be immediately produced by prussic acid, but never unless given in such doses as to occasion difficulty of breathing.*

A defect in calorification and sanguification may exist, in a slight degree, in an early stage of the disease, and not become the most obvious characteristic till the last. Before any profuse alvine evacuations had taken place, I have, in several instances, observed a coldness of the hands and feet, a blueness of the under eyelid, and a preternaturally dark color of the blood drawn from the arm. In this stage also, Dr.

* Am. Jour. of Med. Sci. Vol. xi. p. 501, from a European Journal.—Dr. Hartwig, who made this discovery, blackened the blood by different acids, but could not, it appears, produce this effect by *nitric* acid.—Ibid. I have, however, ascertained by experiment, that nitric acid *does* render the sanguineous coloring matter black as seen by *reflected* (though not as seen by transmitted) light. Has this distinction between the reflected and transmitted light been made by those who have experimented on the blood? By other experiments on blood more nearly normal, I have proved, that the effect of saline substances on the blood at one temperature, cannot be inferred from experiments made at another; and that the blackening of crassamentum by hot water, is not, as has been asserted, dependent on the extraction of its saline matters; and also, that the change of color produced in the sanguineous coloring matter by heat, is not the result of the extrication of oxygen or any other gas. For these experiments, vide Transactions of the Medical Society of the State of New-York, vol. ii. p. 181.

Baird found the heat of the skin below the healthy standard. Dr. McIntyre notices a slightly discolored state of the under eyelid, as among the most frequent premonitory symptoms. Others have observed, that the dark color of the skin frequently prevails as a premonitory symptom from one to ten days, whilst there is no peculiarity in the evacuations.

That no other disease effects so remarkable a change in the composition, color and temperature of the blood, must be admitted; also that these alterations are disproportionate to the amount of alvine evacuations, whether we compare different cases of this disease, or this disease with others; although, neither the physiology of respiration, the chemistry of normal blood, nor the chemical pathology of Cholera, is so complete, as to justify any positive opinion as to the precise time, nor any complete theory of the manner, in which these changes commence. Indeed, the pathogeny of most diseases is obscure; and pathology seldom detects the first links in the chain of morbid phenomena. In Cholera, it can hardly be considered more fortunate with respect to some of the subsequent ones. There is no complete theory; and I do not offer the above as such.

Fortunately for mankind, Hahnemann has discovered a law of cure which is not based upon pathological speculations. The want of such a law and of any reliable guide, is the real cause of the want of unanimity and I may say the uncertainty, confusion and anarchy, that prevails in the allopathic school.

These have, in the case of no disease, been more conspicuous than in relation to Cholera, and never more so than at the present time.

CHAPTER II.

ÆTIOLOGY,

ESPECIALLY WITH REFERENCE TO THE PREDISPOSING AND OCCASIONAL CAUSES.

PRELIMINARY ÆTIOLOGICAL REMARKS.

The peculiar cause of the Cholera is unknown. Hahnemann, and some other learned men, have thought it to be probably an animated miasm. It seems frequently to manifest some self-moving power, or at least to be capable of diffusing itself and of travelling, independently of transportation by human beings, or by the wind. Whatever be its nature, whether animalcular, gaseous, or electrical, it must possess extreme tenuity to escape detection; and its terrific potency is well calculated to rebuke the scepticism of those who sneer at the evidence of efficiency in attenuated medicines, and in everything not cognizable by their senses of sight, smell, hearing, taste or touch.

But as the nature of the cause of Cholera is involved in obscurity, and as I shall under the head of infection, give some views in relation to its propagation, I shall here limit myself to its *predisposing* and *occasional causes*, as related to the pathological phenomena above considered.

If we say that Cholera is attended with great depression of the vital forces, and that the predisposing causes are such as depress these forces or produce general debility, we make a statement which is, to a certain extent and in a certain sense, correct, but is deficient in definite meaning, and but partially true in any sense. If it were strictly and generally true, we should expect that individuals who were robust and muscular, and at the middle period of life, would, cæteris paribus, have a comparative immunity from the disease. But this is far from being the fact. The views about to be presented, not only refer to a definite function, but to a class of correspondences which are more marked in Cholera than in any other disease.

There are many reasons for believing, that during the prevalence of Cholera there is some wide-spread miasm or other aërial epidemic influence tending to diminish the aëration of the blood. We have perhaps some indirect evidence, in the nearly simultaneous prevalence of certain diseases in which the blood is similarly affected, though in an inferior degree. Is there not in many places, either antecedently, or subsequently, an increased prevalence of certain diseases which are attended with dark blood, such as measles, and typhus and other malignant and occasionally anomalous fevers? For weeks and months before the acknowledged incursion of Cholera, there are frequently cases of disease which in these respects nearly resemble it, as I am convinced by my own observations and those of many other physicians.

But to give more satisfactory proof of this connexion between Cholera and respiration, I shall proceed to examine, whether the history of Cholera does not present a class of etiological facts, which, considered in connexion with the results of experiments that have been made on respiration, without any reference to Cholera, tend to confirm the foregoing views with regard to one of its principal, if not essential features.

ATMOSPHERIC HEAT.

The influence of external *heat* on respiration was discovered by Crawford. His experiments and those of others have satisfactorily shown, that the quantity of oxygen consumed and of carbonic acid produced during respiration, is less as the temperature of the air is more elevated. All who have experimented on the subject, with but one exception, have detected this influence of temperature. Crawford found that a Guinea pig, confined in air at the temperature of 55° Fah., consumed double the quantity of oxygen which it did in air at 104°. In the case of human respiration, Lavoisier and Seguin ascertained, that the quantity at 57° is to that at 82° as 1344 is to 1210. Delaroche, in his last series of experiments, made the average ratio about as six to five at the temperatures tried by him. He found, that by elevation of temperature, the production of carbonic acid was diminished, and the absorption of oxygen diminished in a still higher ratio. More recently Dr. Edwards has examined the effect of different seasons, and found that the *long-continued* actions of heat and cold affect the respiration as a vital function; the oxygen consumed being less in summer, even when the air in which the animal is confined at the time, is of the same density and temperature. Moreover, from the experiments above related respecting the influence of sudden changes of temperature, as well as from the known effect of temperature on density, it appears to me evident, that its physical changes between winter and summer, must be such as to make the immediate influence of heat conspire with its gradual physiological effects, and render the consumption in winter and summer still more disproportionate. The influence of heat in diminishing the consumption of oxygen may be considered as established.

On the other hand, few facts are better established, than the influence of hot climates and the warm season of the year in predisposing to Cholera. The epidemic in 1817—which subsequently spread over a considerable portion of the globe, and arrived here in 1832—commenced in summer in the hot climate of

Hindostan; it has generally, in all climates, been much checked if not extinguished by winter; also on cold, elevated mountains. Its ravages in Mexico proved, that it can rise to a great height above the surface of the sea in *warm* climates. In Russia, the southern regions were those where it spread most widely and rapidly; and those towns which it entered at the end of autumn, suffered but slightly.* It is no evidence against these views, that it lingered in winter, in some of the highly-heated, ill-ventilated and filthy rooms of that country. Even in Persia and Asia Minor, the influence of winter on epidemic cholera was manifest during several successive years.† This influence of temperature has been confirmed by the progress of the disease on the western continent. In 1832, it commenced in spring, and until the autumnal cold, nothing impeded its rapid march or changed its malignant character. Both were restored by the heat of the ensuing spring; and again suspended by winter. In its second tour in 1849, the influence of temperature was manifest. At the Quarantine on Staten Island, it disappeared at the commencement of the first severe cold of January; and even the cold of December was sufficient to arrest it in the city of New-York, which had been slightly inoculated. We owe our present immunity, our respite, to cold. The epidemic in New-Orleans in 1848, prevailed in its greatest intensity when the thermometer

* Report of M. Moreau de Jonnes.
† Report of the French Academy.

stood at its greatest height, and disappeared when the weather became sufficiently cold.

BECOMING CHILLED BY COLD AIR OR BY COLD BATHING.

It is remarkable, that the transient application of a cold sufficient to produce a certain degree of *chilliness*, produces the same effect as long-continued heat, both in relation to Cholera and to respiration.

It is known that becoming chilled greatly increases the liability to Cholera.

Dr. Edwards found that in the animals on which he experimented, as well as in man, the becoming chilled, effected more than a mere transient reduction of temperature; it actually weakened the heat-producing power. This was proved by its requiring a longer time for the animal to recover its warmth after the second exposure than after the first. He states also, that in a severe winter, in which the Seine was frozen, a young man in attempting to cross it, broke the ice and fell into the water; but being strong and active, he succeeded in getting out. His health did not suffer; but for three days he had a continual sensation of cold. This was not so simple an affection of the nervous system as a mere prolongation of a strong impression, but it was an alteration of function—a diminution of the heat-producing power.*

* Vide—Influence of Physical Agents on Life, by W. F. Edwards, M.D., F.R.S.

We hardly need refer to such high authority for facts like this last. Most persons are conscious, after being excessively chilled and then warmed by the heat of a fire, that on returning immediately into the cold air, they for a while experience more chilliness than at the first period of the previous exposure. It is unphilosophical to refer these first effects of being chilled (or taking cold) to check of perspiration; for perspiration, as connected with the evaporation which attends it, is physically a cooling process; and the check of it would immediately produce warmth, were it not for the operation of the principle above stated.

It is well to add here a word of *application*, at a time when many exaggerate the advantages, and overlook the dangers, of powerful *baths*. This delusion will have its victims, especially during the prevalence of Cholera. Cleanliness may, and it should be preserved, without making any strong or durable impression, either of heat or cold. This is the true criterion of safe ablution. In addition to the danger of excessive bathing to the community in general, there is one which should not be overlooked by those who are under Homœopathic treatment, either for the cure of disease or for preparing their systems to resist the epidemic. Strongly-impressing baths disturb the action of remedies. Hahnemann justly considered their present effect as analogous to that of large doses of drugs, and their frequent repetition, as tending to retard the cure of chronic diseases. I shall, under another head, give some rules for bathing, but at present advert to other predisposing causes of Cholera.

THE NIGHT SEASON

It has been ascertained, that the quantity of carbonic acid produced, is less in the *night* than in the day-time. Whether this depends directly on the absence of the sun or not, is not certainly known. From the well established relation between the aëration of the blood and animal heat, considered in connexion with the opinion which Dr. Edwards' experiments led him to entertain, that there is less animal heat evolved during sleep, we may conclude that sleep contributes in some measure to the defect of aëration. Rest may be added, as *moderate* exercise increases oxygenation. But this has no material influence on the value of the above-mentioned fact, except that it tends to confirm the influence of night, the usual season of rest and of sleep. Now it has been frequently stated, that the attacks of Cholera are generally more frequent during the night. At Smyrna, in October, 1831, and in some other places, the mortality, it was said, occurred principally in the night. The French Royal Academy of Medicine stated in their report that the invasion of the disease had generally taken place in the night and towards morning. Now, Dr. Prout found that the carbonic acid in the respired air, reached its minimum at half-past eight in the evening, and remained at the minimum state till half-past three in the morning. As the effects of this defective aëration of the blood, are accumulating during the whole of this period, during which it remains at the minimum state, should we not expect that, in proportion as the influence of night predominated among the causes of the disease, it would manifest itself oftener towards morning? And is not the principle analogous to that on which depends the more wide and rapid extension and the increased severity of Cholera, and some other malignant diseases which are connected, though less remarkably, with a defective aëration of the blood, at the close of that season of the year in which this function is at its minimum? A similar principle is applied in physics, to the explanation of the observed time of maximum temperature both of the day and year.

DEPRESSING PASSIONS, FATIGUE, FASTING AND ALCOHOL.

Dr. Prout ascertained, by direct experiment, that the quantity of carbonic acid produced during respiration is diminished by the *depressing passions*, or even *strong* mental *emotions* of any kind; by *long-continued and violent exercise;* by *fasting;* and by *intemperate habits*, and even the *moderate use of alcoholic liquors*. It is well known, that all these are powerful predisposing causes of epidemic *Cholera*,

The disease has been frequently favored by the fatiguing marches of armies, and the privations which they have suffered; by the existence of poverty with its attendant evils, of excessive labor and scanty food; by violent anger, by the depressing passions, such as the fear of the disease itself; and by intemperate habits, and even the moderate use of alcoholic liquors. The want of success which has generally attended the administration of alcohol in this disease would not of itself be conclusive, but it may have some weight. The foregoing views respecting the causes and nature of epidemic Cholera, and a knowledge of the specific action of alcohol in diminishing the oxygenation of the blood, in all individuals, however temperate and healthy, might have led us to anticipate that its influence in predisposing to this disease, would not be confined to the broken-down drunkard. This inference from theory is confirmed by experience. In relation to that form of the disease, in which at the height of the epidemic in Vienna, it most nearly approximated to the perfect type, and in which the seizure was sudden, the evacuations almost or altogether wanting, the cramps severe, and the fatal termination in most cases in a few hours, it was observed that a middle age, vigor of constitution, and such a use of gin, as had not materially affected it, were predisposing causes.*

* London Lancet, for June 23d, 1832.

The last is a practice which diminishes the aëration of the blood, and the two former are circumstances under which, as has often been shown, such diminution can be tolerated with least impunity. In relation to ardent spirits, as predisposing to this disease, mistakes have arisen from too wide a distinction between *drinking* and *drunkenness*. These mistakes would be corrected by physiological views.

ABSTINENCE FROM ANIMAL FOOD.

Dr. Fyfe proved by experiment, that the carbonic acid was *reduced to nearly one-half by vegetable diet*. Now this is the diet which has predominated in those countries, in those cities, and in those classes of society, in which the disease has been most fatal, whether in Asia, Europe or America. It is true, some physicians have recommended vegetable food during the epidemic, interdicting only unripe vegetables, and a few kinds generally admitted to be peculiarly unwholesome. But this preference for vegetable food must proceed rather from an incorrect theory, and from their experience in other diseases supposed by them to be analogous, than from their experience or that of the world, in this disease.* In the report published by the au-

* Most species of *grain*, however, being more easy of digestion and containing more azote than most other parts of vegetables, make a nearer approximation to animal food, and are hence less injurious than some other vegetable substances.

thority of the French Academy, it is affirmed, that during the Cholera at Calcutta, "those who lived on vegetable substances were first taken off; and that women and children seemed to be spared." I quote the whole passage, as the latter part affords some evidence, that this influence of vegetable food is not, as some have supposed, referable merely to the debility and consequent irritability induced by it.

Moreover, that it was mode of living, and not idiosyncrasy, that rendered the Hindoos so much more liable to the disease than the English residents, may be argued from the fact, that the native soldiers, whose mode of living was more similar to that of the English, enjoyed a similar degree of exemption. Indeed, it was every where observed, that those who subsisted on vegetable food, were selected as the first victims. Perhaps it may be worthy of remark, that the unusual mortality in Paris, where at the least twenty thousand of the inhabitants were carried off in a month, occurred during the season of Lent. Immediately after Easter the virulence of the disease rapidly abated. The proportion of vegetable food is usually great among a French population. May not the severe Cholera of Montreal and New-Orleans, in 1832, be cited as in some degree examples of its influence? On the ensuing spring, the disease, after its winter's sleep, awoke in the Catholic city of Havana, in the season of Lent. It numbered among its victims many of the most respectable and religious citizens, and produced a mortality unprecedented in the history of its ravages in the western hemisphere.* Were these isolated facts, they would merit less regard. But the influence of vegetable food, has been generally observed to predispose to Cholera, and even to epizoötics strongly resembling it; but never, in any instance which I have heard,

* Among other respectable individuals who fell victims, was the Archbishop of Havana. On some days 900 are said to have died out of a population of about 180,000. Not having access, however, to official documents, I extract this from the newspapers, as also the following account of the recommencement of the march of the disease in Louisiana, nearly at the same time. The following is from the Albany Argus of April 15th, 1833. "The Louisiana Republican, printed at Franklin, in the Attakapas region, says that the Cholera has begun to assume, in that quarter, a more formidable appearance. At first, few cases proved fatal, except those which occurred among the colored population; persons of temperate habits were seldom attacked." [This shows the influence of alcohol.] "But of late, citizens *particularly noted* for their temperance have fallen victims." [This shows, perhaps, the combined effects of heat, vegetable diet, and fasting.] The St. Martinsville (Lou.) Courier, of 22d March, gives a similar account of its prevalence in that place and its vicinity. "As it was nearly stationary during the winter, we thought that the salubrity of our situation would preserve us; but within the last three weeks, it appears to have extended its exterminating influence, and we have already to deplore the loss of several respectable inhabitants of our parish, as also a great number of slaves." Now it is worthy of notice, that the 24th of Feb., was the first Sunday in Lent; and it would seem that the extension of its "exterminating influence," commenced about a week afterwards. What intemperance did for the lower and dissolute, did not fasting and vegetable diet contribute to effect for the higher and religious classes? Those who are better acquainted with their habits can judge.

among animals exclusively carnivorous. I need only allude to the epizoötic which prevailed among several species of herbivorous animals in Scotland, and to the mortality among the fowls of Choisi near Paris; to their white alvine discharges; and the dark color assumed by their combs, affording, from their translucence, an index to the color of the blood.

From the effects of vegetable diet and abstinence from food, I must believe, that a fast in either of these senses, during the epidemic, would tend to aggravate the awful calamity which it might be proposed for the purpose of averting; yet, on the other hand, as strong emotions, and especially the depressing passions, have been shown to produce an influence similar to that of fasting, it is evident that a religious frame of mind, a calm and cheerful reliance on Divine Providence, must be among the best preservatives. During the prevalence of Cholera, it should be considered a sacred duty to avoid fasting, except so far as fasting is dictated by want of appetite.

OPPRESSION OF THE DIGESTIVE ORGANS, WITH FOOD INDIGESTIBLE IN QUALITY OR EXCESSIVE IN QUANTITY.

This is another cause of impaired calorific function, as well as of Cholera. During the first stage of a digestion rendered laborious by indigestible food or over-eating, all persons, especially, those of weak digestive powers, are conscious of some degree of chilliness on exposure to cold. This, as Dr. Edwards has explained in the cases before cited, is not merely a simple nervous impression, but an alteration of function, a diminution of the power of generating animal heat.

Now it is known, that excess in eating, even in the case of wholesome food, and the use of indigestible substances, as crude and flatulent vegetables, clams, the meat of young animals, &c., especially by persons of weak digestion, frequently disposes to an attack of Cholera.

CROWDED OR INSUFFICIENTLY VENTILATED ROOMS.

The *air* of *rooms* which are occupied by too many persons, or insufficiently ventilated, diminishes the aëration of the blood and the generation of animal heat, and also predisposes to an attack of Cholera. It is unnecessary to cite any proofs of the former proposition. Air deficient in oxygen and charged with carbonic acid, cannot properly sustain the calorific function. Its effect in predisposing to Cholera, the history of this epidemic sufficiently manifests. The principle here referred to, is distinct from that of infection. When the disease has once entered a room, both principles co-operate. But crowded and ill-ventilated rooms not only conduce to the communication of the disease when once admitted, but they invite it to enter.

The occupants of basements seem, cæteris paribus, to be more liable to the disease. This may be owing to the combined effect of carbonic acid and humidity, and perhaps of the tendency of Cholera miasm to travel into low places. That some of the other circumstances above enumerated, exert on the miasm a physical influence, which conspires with their physiological influence on man, in exciting the disease, is not improbable.

NEGLECT OF PERSONAL CLEANLINESS.

The accumulation of cutaneous filth sustains to respiration, animal heat and the state of the blood, and to Cholera, a relation similar to that of the ten other circumstances above considered: but its influence is less striking. By mechanically obstructing the cutaneous pores, filth must in some measure diminish the aëration of the blood, which is known to be effected in part by the skin. There is here, as in the lungs, an absorption of oxygen and elimination of carbonic acid. There is in man, a cutaneous as well as pulmonary respiration; though it is less remarkable than in frogs and other animals of the order batrachia, which will survive the loss of their lungs longer than that of their skin.

But in man, the obstruction of the cutaneous pores is more important in its relation to the pulmonary than to the cutaneous respiration, or even to the cutaneous perspiration; as was intimated when treating of the effects of being chilled. The liquid transpired could, if suppressed, be chiefly eliminated by the kidneys; but although other evils would ultimately result from this retention, the first morbid effects of obstructing the cutaneous pores, even as it relates to transpiration, seem to relate chiefly to the oxygenating and calorific function.

UNGENERALIZED FACTS.

Among the circumstances which physiologists have found to diminish the quantity of oxygen, there are, in addition to those which have been enumerated, a few others, the influence of which in predisposing to this disease requires further investigation. These are the use of tea; the administration of nitric acid; affecting the system by a course of mercury; and placing the body in a posture which impedes respiration. I am acquainted with no general etiological fact in relation to these, which militates against the foregoing views; and from the evidence above adduced, in relation to agencies similar to these in one of their physiological relations, I believe that persons by taking green tea, nitric acid, blue pills or calomel, would be more liable to Cholera.

On the other hand, among the predisposing causes of Cholera, there are some, whose influence on the consumption of oxygen requires further investigation.

Many cases of Asiatic Cholera have been produced by cathartics. I have known several instances. I might give a plausible explanation by which such facts could be brought under the above law; but I prefer abstaining from all hypothesis.

In the same class of ungeneralized facts, I shall for similar reasons, place the influence of certain changes in the hygrometric, barometric and electrical states of the atmosphere. These are so generally connected, that simultaneous and repeated observations, and a nice discrimination, would be requisite to determine their separate influences even on cholera. In August, 1832, I observed at two different times, a considerable *depression* of the barometer and elevation of the dewpoint, and at both times, there was, I believe, a sudden and considerable increase of the disease both in Albany and Schenectady. As the epidemic, having commenced at different times in these two neighboring cities, was not in the same stage, these simultaneous changes must be attributed to a meteorological influence. If humidity was the cause, humidity as detected by the hygrometer, seemed to have more influence than rain. That the effect depended partly on an electrical change preceding a storm, is not improbable. Finally, there are many agents whose influences both on the consumption of oxygen and the production of Cholera are alike unknown. If, as appears from numerous considerations above stated, there is any law connecting these influences, then experiments for determining the effect of these agents on respiration, might lead to important practical applications in relation to the prevention, if not to the treatment of the disease. In applying the results, however, regard should be had to the difference between the immediate and remote effects on respiration; these are frequently opposite.

RECAPITULATION.

Without the aid of any mere hypothesis, I have shown, that there is a remarkable correspondence between certain classes of physiological and ætiological facts, in relation to Cholera. This correspondence is interesting on account of the dependence of animal heat and the florid color of arterial blood on respiration, considered in connexion with the fact, that in an advanced state of dangerous cases of every variety of this disease, and in an early stage of the severer varieties, no pathological phenomena are more constant, than a dark color of the blood and a temperature below the normal standard.

As a large proportion of the occasional or predisposing causes are in a great measure under the control of man, a statement of these and of the scientific evidence of their influence, will tend to inspire hope and promote safety.

I have shown that physiology concurs with general experience, in proving the following to be the principal predisposing causes of Cholera: viz., 1st, *hot climates and hot seasons*; 2d, *becoming chilled by cold air or by cold bathing;* 3d, *the night season;* 4th, *fear and other depressing emotions*; 5th, *violent and excessively fatiguing exercise;* 6th, *total fasting*, i. e. *abstinence* from *all food;* 7th, *partial fasting*, i. e. *abstinence from animal food;* 8th, *oppressing the stomach with food indigestible in quality or excessive in quantity;* 9th, *the moderate as well as intemperate use of alcoholic drinks;* 10th, *crowded or insufficiently ventilated rooms;* and 11th, *neglect of personal cleanliness.*

The order in which these are enumerated, has no reference to their relative potency, but to their natural affinities.

CHAPTER III.

DOCTRINE OF INFECTION

WITH REFERENCE TO THIS DISEASE.

ERROR OF THE PREVALENT DOCTRINE.

An opinion extensively entertained by the profession, is, that there is a certain class of diseases, including small pox, measles, scarlatina and hooping cough, which an individual may take on coming near a patient affected with them, although the intermediate air be pure; and that there is another class of diseases, including plague, yellow fever, typhus fever, dysentery and cholera, which an individual cannot take, unless the intermediate air between him and the patient is impure, and that he takes these from the air, and not by any specific poison derived either directly or indirectly from the patient. The former class of diseases, they denominate contagious; the latter class, infectious.

But in both cases, the disease *is* communicated through the air, and in consequence of its contamination; and in both cases by a specific poison, else the same kind of disease as that with which the first patient was affected would not be reproduced. These classes of disease, when communicated through the air, differ, not in the *principle* or *mode* of communication, but in the quantity or *dose* of the poison, which is requisite for reproducing the disease.

The terms contagion and infection, as now extensively used in a technical sense, serve only to conceal the want of precise ideas, and the defects of a false mode of reasoning. Whence the disputes and hesitation of learned academies, and of the medical world generally, in relation to this subject? In my opinion, this confusion, disagreement and indecision arise from not viewing the subject in a mathematical point of view, that is, in its relation to the science of *quantity*. The popular mind is prone to inquire about the *existence* of certain *things* or entities, rather than their quantitative relations. It asks, is there infection in this disease or in that? It does not think to inquire, whether there is *more* or *less* infecting power. It does not suspect that this is the only difference in many diseases in regard to their power of propagating themselves. The medical mind, perhaps from deficiency of mathematical training, is extensively infected with this same intellectual vice. Physicians, instead of recognizing degrees in the infecting power, generally found their distinctions on modes and media of transmission. Again, instead of recognizing a great diversity, as they would if they had hit on the true principle of distinction, they assume that all except a few diseases are incommunicable under any circumstances; and through those that they acknowledge capable of propagation, they arbitrarily draw a single line, and denominate the whole group on one side of that line contagious, and the whole group on the other side infectious. They have not yet perceived that what they call infection, considered as a property of the disease, is merely the contagious property in less intensity. For convenience, I shall use the terms infection and infectious in their most comprehensive sense, which embraces all modes of communication.

INDEFINITENESS OF THE PROBLEM.

To ask whether Asiatic Cholera is infectious, is like asking whether diluted alcohol is an intoxicating drink. Is diluted alcohol an intoxicating drink, or is it not? Does not every one perceive, that for the solution of this problem, the requisite data are not given in the question? It is indefinite in three respects; viz., first, as to the degree of dilution of the alcohol; secondly, as to the quantity to be taken; and thirdly, as to the susceptibility of the drinker to its intoxicating influence. One part of alcohol diluted with ten thousand parts of water, is not an intoxicating drink, in any quantity which the stomach can retain: one part of alcohol diluted with one hundred parts of water, is not an intoxicating drink, unless taken in enormous quantities, or by persons highly susceptible.

The problem, in regard to the infectiousness of Cholera, is of a similar nature, and is to be solved by a reference to precisely the same three conditions, viz. dilution, quantity and susceptibility.

INFLUENCE OF DILUTION.

If several Cholera patients should at the same time occupy the same small and ill-ventilated room, the air of that room would, after some time, become so charged with the miasm, as to be capable of communicating Cholera to other occupants, provided that by their constitution, their state of health, their neglect of regimen and of prophylactic remedies, they possessed a certain degree of susceptibility to the disease. To them, the disease would be infectious, in this concentrated state of the morbific miasm. On the other hand, if there were only one patient in a large and well-ventilated-room, the respiration of its air during the same length of time, and by individuals having the same predisposition, might be perfectly safe, and would certainly be attended with little danger as compared with that in the small, close and crowded room above-mentioned. What, in a more concentrated state, was a poison, becomes comparatively innoxious by dilution. If we admit the possibility of taking Cholera under these last circumstances—if we say that even in such a room it is possible that Cholera may to some persons prove infectious, our statement is liable to be misunderstood and misapplied. One will say, Cholera is then infectious, like small-pox. This would be a gross exaggeration, and one which it is important to prevent; inasmuch as it would deter many from giving the requisite attention to the sick, and also excite, among those not yet attacked, an alarm that would increase their susceptibility. The miasm of small-pox is one that operates in a much more diluted state than that of Cholera, and requires no peculiar susceptibility except that naturally possessed by persons who have not been vaccinated. Such persons by going near a small-pox patient, even in a large and well-ventilated room, would be in great danger of taking the disease. The danger of this in case of exposure to a Cholera patient under the same circumstances, would be comperatively trifling.

Again, even the miasm of small-pox can, by diffusion in the open air, be so diluted, as to lose entirely its poisonous property, and become incapable of producing the disease. Still more easily does this take place in case of the Cholera Miasm. We have seen, that for weeks it confined itself to the hospitals at Staten-Island, without passing beyond their common enclosure to affect the village in which they are situated. In 1853—54 there have been similar instances in the same locality.

For security from infection by Cholera miasm, it must have a certain degree of dilution. Among the *practical applications* to be made of this doctrine, we may mention the importance of ventilation, of using as large rooms as possible for Cholera patients, and allowing as few patients as possible to be confined in the same room. Ventilation and washing are the only requisites for the purification of rooms which have been occupied by Cholera patients. There is no evidence that chlorine or chloride of lime has the slightest influence on this infecting miasm itself; and the fumigation of the sick-room would be decidedly prejudical, both to the patient and his attendants. In addition to the direct deleterious action of the gas on the system, it would interfere with the salutary action of medicines and prophylactics.

INFLUENCE OF DOSE.

Having considered the influence of dilution, I shall proceed to that of *quantity*. If any poison is diluted to that degree in which it just begins to lose its power of acting as a poison, in a certain dose, it will still act as a poison in a larger dose, or (what is nearly equivalent in practical effect) in numerous and frequently repeated doses, the aggregate of which is a very large quantity.

The Cholera miasm observes the same law. A room, occupied by Cholera patients, may be so large and well-ventilated, that a susceptible individual might be perfectly safe in it for three hours, but not for thirty. During the latter period, he would inhale ten times as much air slightly impregnated with the miasm. Allopathic physicians have frequently seen the mischievous and even fatal effects of mercury and arsenic in what *they* call small doses, administered by them for a considerable length of time.

Still there is nothing on earth which is a *poison*, irrespective of concentration and dose. We cannot consider the Deity as the Author of any thing which is poisonous, i. e. destructive, in its very essence. Read the impressive language of Hahnemann. "When He, the All-bountiful, created iron, He left it to the free choice of the children of men, to fashion it either into the deadly dagger, or the peaceful ploughshare, to slay or to support their race. Ah, how much happier for them, did they employ all His gifts for good! So would they fulfil His will and the end of their being. We cannot charge an all-loving Providence with the crimes, that men have committed in abusing the administration of terribly powerful drugs, by giving them in enormous doses, and in improper cases."

Such were the elevated sentiments that animated the man, who will, in all future times, be remembered as the first discoverer of a method, by which the noxious properties of the most virulent poisons may be removed, whilst their curative properties are retained or heightened. The success of this pharmaceutic method depends greatly on that minute division which is effected by a certain diluting process; yet the first object in the mind of its discoverer was the reduction of dose. He aimed to diminish the quantity of a crude allopathic drug to such a degree, that it should cease to be a poison, that is, become a medicine fit for homœopathic use. I have been insensibly led to speak of this method, when considering the effect of inhaling a greater or less quantity of air impregnated with Cholera miasm.

Whether Cholera is or is not infectious, depends not only on the degree in which the air is impregnated with the miasm, but upon the quantity of the air inhaled, and consequently upon the length of time during which it is continuously respired.

I will make *another application* of these views relative to the latter topic. Wherever it is practicable, there should be a provision for the occasional relief of *nurses;* so that no one should be required to spend the whole day, much less day and night, in the sick-chamber.

For making such a desirable arrangement, the homœopathic system offers peculiar advantages. In the first place, homœopathic families will have fewer cases of Cholera; secondly, these cases will be of much shorter duration, i. e. will sooner terminate in health; and thirdly, they will require less nursing in proportion to their number and duration. Every family which has enjoyed homœopathic practice, knows what an amount of nurse-labor is dispensed with by avoiding external applications, to say nothing of evacuants, which in case of Cholera the disease itself often supplies, as if to give, at the same time, a specimen and a reproof, of allopathy carried to perfection.

INFLUENCE OF SUSCEPTIBILITY.

But not only does Cholera fail to be infectious, unless there is a sufficient concentration of the poison in the air, and a sufficient quantity of this air respired; but it also fails to be infectious, unless there is a peculiar predisposition or *susceptibility* in the person exposed. Some possess an immunity, from the very nature of their constitutions, others by the good state of their health at the time, others by the judicious regulation of their diet and regimen, and others in consequence of having taken the homœopathic prophylactics, i. e. preventive medicines.

What I have to say hereafter in regard to the success of prophylactic and therapeutic measures, is calculated to confirm the confidence and hopes of the homœopathic members of the community; and what I have said in regard to infection, is also calculated to allay anxiety. When the public are apprized, that, in the last travel of the Cholera, the first place in which it appeared on this continent, was not in any filthy street, of any large city, but in a hospital into which Cholera patients had been recently introduced, it will be difficult to persuade them, that the vicinity of those already affected with Cholera, has not some influence in propagating the disease. The anxiety which such a fact is calculated to excite, is not allayed by the disputes of the faculty in regard to the question whether the disease is, or is not contagious, nor by any distinctive names, expressing merely the modes of communication. The true solace is to be derived from a consideration of the various degrees of infecting power, and the feebleness of that of Cholera; and the true security is to be derived from an examination and application of the principles, on which this infecting power is still farther enfeebled, so as to become scarcely appreciable, and from those prophylactic measures which diminish or remove individual susceptibility.

It is probable, that almost all diseases are more or less communicable to individuals who have a peculiar susceptibility to their respective influences. Some of these diseases, as small-pox, are generated by the reception of inconceivably minute doses of the morbid product. Small-pox, again, is an example of a disease which requires no special susceptibility; none which is not naturally possessed by almost all persons previously to vaccination; whereas a majority escape Cholera, even when they are most fully exposed to it, and pay no special attention to diet or regimen.

In the case of cholera, as well as of most other diseases, the liability to infection depends vastly more upon the peculiar susceptibility of the individual, than upon the degree of exposure. When Cholera is introduced into a city, a majority of its inhabitants may have symptoms which mark its presence in the atmosphere; but only a small proportion usually take the disease, however intimate their communication with the sick; and of those who do become affected with it, there is a large majority who have had no obvious and direct communication with persons laboring under the disease.

ROUTES AND MODES IN WHICH THE CHOLERA TRAVELS.

In its progress from one country to another, and from city to city, it oftener selects the great thoroughfares of men, and especially rivers. Its preference of low situations, and especially of the shores of rivers and other bodies of water, appears however not to be entirely owing to human intercourse. In 1832, I observed that nearly all the cases at the commencement of the epidemic in Schenectady, were for some time in a retired part of the town near the Mohawk, a river not used for navigation. At other times, the disease travels across dry regions, and seems to pass from city to city, independently of human intercourse. Cholera, then travels by two methods; viz., with men as vehicles, and without any obvious and visible vehicles of transportation: - it sometimes goes, at other times it is carried.

During its prevalence in any part of a country or of a city, some degree—more or less slight—of a widely diffused *epidemic influence*, is usually manifested, by a tendency to diseases somewhat similar, provided the season of the year is favorable to the spread of cholera.

As to quarantine regulations, we can rarely expect

from them more than some postponement of the invasion. Even this will justify their rigorous enforcement. The disease is propagated partly, though not exclusively, by infection.

CHAPTER IV.

HYGIENE AND PROPHYLAXIS.

ARTICLES WHICH SHOULD NOT BE USED BY PERSONS WHO ARE TAKING HOMŒOPATHIC MEDICINES, EITHER DURING THE PREVALENCE OF CHOLERA OR AT OTHER TIMES.

1st. Raw vegetables—such as celery, lettuce, &c.;

2d. Unripe, or sour fruits, and acids in general;

3d. Food which has any medicinal qualities—such as onions and tomatoes, and bread prepared with soda;

4th. Coffee, green tea, and distilled and fermented liquors;

5th. Condiments (except salt), as vinegar, pickles, pepper, spices and mustard;

6th. Camphor, hartshorn, cathartics, herb-teas, and other medicines (whether external or internal) except those prescribed by the physician;

7th. Tobacco in great quantities, especially by chewing; and in any quantity unless the individual has been long accustomed to it.

None of the forbidden articles (except coffee, and camphor, and other medicines), need to be suddenly and totally abandoned, if the individual has been long accustomed to them. In that case, he may, unless forbidden by his physician, use them, though in great moderation. Great and sudden changes in regard to the use of condiments, should not be made after the epidemic has actually commenced in the place. Let the reform commence earlier.

HYGIENIC RULES IMPORTANT TO BE OBSERVED BY PERSONS IN GENERAL DURING THE PREVALENCE OF CHOLERA, AND USEFUL AT ALL OTHER TIMES.*

1st. Use warm clothing, and in cool or changeable weather, flannel; but put a cotton or silk garment under it, unless you have been accustomed to flannel next the skin.

2d. Avoid taking cold, or becoming chilled.

3d. Use no cold, nor hot, nor even tepid baths; but use cool baths, those which feel like a summer breeze, or sponge the body with water of such a temperature. This, with different individuals and different modes of using the water, may range from 75° to 80° Fahrenheit.

4th. Remain in the water not longer than a minute; and wash and wipe yourself dry as soon as possible; and if in the least chilly, put on extra clothing.

* The imperative form is used here for brevity.

Use this ablution once a week, or twice in summer, and wash the feet and other more sweaty parts of the body daily.

5th. Endeavor to encourage good temper, hope and cheerfulness, in yourself and others.

6th. Use moderate and even active exercise, but avoid great fatigue.

7th. Avoid all kinds of fasting, when there is appetite.*

8th. Let the diet consist partly of animal food, and partly of good bread or some other preparation of wheat flour.† Use a good proportion of fresh beef, mutton, venison, or fowls, and, if it agrees with the stomach, soup made of one of these meats. Fish, eggs, good milk, butter, sugar, and molasses, are not hurtful to persons in general, when used in moderation, and with a due proportion daily of some of the meats above-mentioned.

9th. Avoid all indigestible food, every thing which you have found to oppress your stomach, whether it be cabbage, turnip, or other succulent vegetables, and especially fibrous vegetables and fibrous fruits, as some kinds of radishes and pine-apples, also fresh bread, rich pastry, old or toasted cheese, meat too fatty, veal or other young meats, sausages, pork, geese, lobsters, shell-fish, eels or other fish which

* I will not deny that any man has a right to punish himself by abstaining from hurtful luxuries; but he has no right to punish himself by injuring his health.

† This last, possessing considerable azote, has some chemical similarity to animal food.

have not both fins and scales. The articles enumerated in this paragraph are of doubtful character for most dyspeptics at all times, and for most persons when Cholera prevails.

10th. Eat with moderation: take care not to overload the stomach with food of any kind.

11th. Masticate the food throughly. If possible observe regular and early hours for eating and sleeping. Avoid late suppers: but if compelled to defer the evening meal till a late hour, eat sparingly.

12th. Drink water, cocoa, pure unspiced chocolate, toast-water, barley-water, or weak black tea.

13th. Avoid as far as possible all alcoholic drinks, whether distilled or fermented, but especially the former. Use neither coffee nor green tea.

14th. Keep your room properly ventilated, but in such a manner as not to expose yourself to currents of air when sitting still.

15th. Do not continue long in small rooms that are crowded with people.

16th. If practicable, avoid sleeping in basements, or with many persons in the same room.

Peculiarities of constitution and inveterate habits, and the disadvantages of making great and sudden changes after the commencement of the epidemic, will justify some modification in the above rules by some individuals. In food, some concessions must be made to taste.

PROPHYLACTICS.

The homœopathic *preventives* of Cholera are *Cuprum-metallicum*, and *Veratrum-album*, prepared according to the homœopathic method, and taken alternately in doses of two or three pellets once or twice a week. The globules may be placed on the tongue, and allowed to dissolve in the mouth, and then swallowed.

Wherever it is practicable, a homœopathic physician should be consulted; as one of these remedies would in some cases be preferable to the other. He could decide which.

The method which Hahnemann recommended, and which many employed with success, was to take globules medicated with the 30th dilution of *Cuprum*, then wait one week, and take the similarly medicated globules of the 30th of *Veratrum*; then after a week, the *Cuprum*, and so on. Others have used, with similar success, the third dilution of each, at intervals of half a week. This may be used by those who cannot obtain the thirtieth; but let no one venture upon the use of the copper of the drug stores, nor the crude colored tincture of Veratrum, even of the homœopathic pharmacies.

To those who are not very strict in their homœopathic regimen, it might be well to take each medicine once a week, i. e. alternately at intervals of three or four days. Take the medicine in the morning on rising, an hour before breakfast; or, if at another time, take nothing in the mouth, except pure water, within an hour after taking the medicine.

When a family is to be protected, we might dissolve five or six pellets of the 12th of Veratrum in a gill of clean cold water, and give each member one, two or three tea-spoonfuls, according to the age. Then after waiting three days, use the thirtieth of Cuprum in the same dose and manner; then wait three days, and give the thirtieth of Veratrum in the same dose and manner. Afterwards alternate the thirtieth of each in solution as before described, and at the same intervals. I advise commencing with the Veratrum, because Cholera oftener requires Veratrum, at least in the male sex. Camphor is too transient in its action to be of any use as a prophylactic: besides it would interfere with other medicines. Persons who may be so circumstanced as to think it best to carry it in their pockets, to have it ready in case of attack, should keep it very tightly corked, and, unless attacked, should not use it, even by smelling, when they have been taking a prophylactic.

In 1832, prophylactics were thought to have saved thousands; and some denied that any who had employed them had fallen victims to the disease. I have evidence, though not in the circle of my own practice, that in this city in 1849, there were some results not corroborative of the latter statement, —a statement from which some might presume, that there was complete safety in relying on preventives, even when selected without reference to the peculiar tendencies of each individual. But I am confident that a discriminating treatment of premonitory symptoms, according to the principles and practice recommended in this book was invariably preventive of any fatal attack.

CHAPTER V.

HISTORY OF TREATMENT,

OR

STATISTICAL PROOFS OF THE SUCCESS OF HOMŒOPATHY IN CHOLERA.

PRELIMINARY REMARKS.

A vast number of remedies and modes of allopathic treatment have enjoyed ephemeral reputation, have been lauded, rejected, revived, and again rejected. This may be partly explained by the fact, that medicines and methods employed toward the close of the epidemic in any place, acquire an undue reputation, because the disease is usually at that period less malignant and fatal. The physician not appreciating this, publishes his specific in good faith ; but it utterly fails with those who subsequently try it in a different place, in any stage of the epidemic in which nature is not nearly competent to the cure. There is no plan of treatment agreed upon, even by one-fourth of the allopathic physicians, and very little confidence in allopathic Cholera practice in general, among most of the best informed of that school. An able allopathic author who practised in 1831 and 1832, in England, where homœopathy was then unknown, says, "If the balance could be fairly struck, and the exact truth ascertained, I question whether we should find that the average mortality from Cholera in this country, was any way disturbed by our craft. Excepting always the cases in which preliminary diarrhœa was checked, just as many, though not perhaps the very same individuals, would, probably, have survived, had no medication whatever been practised." *

A friend asks me—How will you treat the Cholera? I answer, homœopathically. I perceive he almost trembles as the thought, provided he is a new convert, and one unacquainted with the homœopathic history of this disease. I endeavor to remove his solicitude, by assuring him that there is no method of treating Cholera which can be compared with Hahnemann's. Has it ever been tried? This question is a very reasonable one. Thousands of Americans will ask it, at a time when the Cholera is approaching them, in a form as virulent as was ever known in Europe or America, if we can judge from the loss of one half the patients, even in private practice, by the European and American allopathists.

* Lectures on the Principles and Practise of Physic; delivered at King's College, London, by Thomas Watson, M. D. p. 828.

I will let statistics answer this question and show the relative results. Whence the horror which the name of this disease awakens? It comes from the deplorable failure of allopathic treatment.

Let no one trust his life to any vaunted method of cure, which has been tried only by a few scores of patients, and by one or two physicians. The homœopathic method has has been tried on many thousands of cholera patients, and with similar success in different countries.

As ratios obtained from large numbers are more reliable for showing the true average, and as the epidemic of 1831—1832 and that of 1849 are those in which the greater number of cases have occurred, and in relation to which more facts can be presented, I shall confine myself chiefly to them.

Some our allopathic brethren, as if conscious of the weakness of their system on the broad field of extensive statistics, are at present restricting themselves to a guerilla warfare. When a single death occurs among the patients of a homœopathic physician, it is noised abroad as something remarkable. But if any one is desirous of knowing the true relative value of the two systems, he must examine the subject on a broader scale. He must consider the number which homœopathy cures, in his own city or neighborhood, and throughout the world, and the average relative results of the two methods of treatment.

THE CHOLERA EPIDEMIC OF 1831—1832.

In 1832 there were in this city including Bellevue 5232 cases, of which 2031 died; i. e. nearly one out of every 2½ or 2⅗, or in round numbers, nearly 2 out of 5. Of persons treated at their homes, there were 2859 cases, of whom 937 died; i. e. about one in every 3 persons attacked. In the hospitals, including Bellevue, there were 2373 cases, and 1094 deaths; i. e. nearly one half died. Such were the best results that could be obtained here by allopathic skill.

In Europe, in 1831—1832, this disease, under allopathic treatment, was still more fatal. In the allopathic hospitals of Italy and France, in 21 of which I have seen the ratio of deaths stated, the average of the ratios gives 63 deaths out of every 100 patients.

The only treatment which proved itself worthy of any confidence, was the homœopathic. It is not denied by allopathists themselves, that it was the great success that attended the homœopathic treatment of Cholera in Europe, that gave this system the most powerful impulse that it has ever received. Dr. Balfour of Edinburgh, who is opposed to the system, writes to Dr. Forbes from Vienna in 1836, in the following words: "During the first appearance of Cholera here, the practice of homœopathy was first introduced; and Cholera, when it came again, renewed the favorable impulse previously given, as it was through Dr. Fleischmann's successful treatment of this disease, that the restrictive laws were removed, and homœopathists obtained leave to practise and dispense medicines in Austria. Since that time their number has increased more than threefold in Vienna and its provinces." He also says: "No young physician settling in Austria—excluding government officers—can hope to make his bread, unless at least prepared to treat homœopathically, if requested."[1]

Let us compare the results of the two systems in the same city. In Vienna, there were 4500 patients treated allopathically; of whom 1360 died. There were 581 treated homœopathically; of whom only 49 died. This give 31 per cent. of deaths under the former, and only 8 per cent. under the latter.

Dr. Quin of London has given a table of the results of the treatment of ten different homœopathic physicians. The worst result under any of these physicians was, the death of only one-fifth of his patients, whilst four-fifths were saved. The best result obtained by any one of these physicians was the saving of 40 out of every 41, or losing 3 out of 125, this being the number of cases which he treated. This physician was Dr. Weith of Vienna. These cures were made at a time when this pestilence was prevailing in that city in its greatest intensity, and baffling all the skill of allopathic physicians.

The statements of this venerable man can be relied on. He is above suspicion. He had no party prejudices to mislead him; no professional interests to advance. Though he had taken the degree of Doctor of medicine, his profession was that of a minister of religion. But when he beheld his fellow-citizens doomed to destruction, his feelings as a man, and his principles as a christian, impelled him to stretch forth his arm for their relief. He had just become convinced of the truth of the homœopathic doctrine, and of its practical importance. It was distressing to him, to be continually called to the death-beds of persons who might have been saved by homœopathy, but were perishing in spite of allopathy. His spirit was stirred within him, and he resolved to suspend in part and for a time his functions as the spiritual guide of his people, and devote himself to their temporal salvation. He acted as a true disciple of Him, who delighted in saving not only the souls but the lives of men.

The efforts of Dr. Weith were crowned with a success fully justifying the expectations which he had been led to entertain by the success of other homœopathic physicians in this same epidemic.

The remedies which he employed, were *Phosphoric-acid*, *Veratrum*, *Cuprum*, Tincture of *Camphor*, and under some circumstances, lavements of ice-water.

Of the 1093 patients, treated by the ten homœopathic physicians, 998 were saved, and only 95 lost. Thus the average proportion of deaths was only one to 11½, or 2 out of 23 patients, whilst 21 out of 23 patients were saved. The results above stated were chiefly obtained at Vienna, in Moravia, Bohemia and Hungary, during the epidemic of 1831 and 1832.

Dr. Rath, who had been sent, in April, 1832, by order of the king of Bavaria, to collect authentic information respecting the results of the homœopathic treatment of the Cholera, reported officially the several results of the treatment of 14 homœopathic physicians at Prague, in Moravia, in Hungary and at Vienna. The total number of cases which he reported was 1269; cures 1184, deaths 85.

In Russia and Austria, and at Berlin and Paris, there were 3017 cases treated homœopathically; of which 2753 were cured, and only 264 died; i. e. only about one in 11½ died. On an average more than 10 out of 11 were cured.

Hon. Alexis Eustaphieve, the Russian Consul General, has given the results obtained by homœopathic treatment in various parts of the Russian Empire in 1830 and 1831. Of 70 patients treated in two places, all were cured. The total result was, that of 1270 patients, 1162 were saved, and only 108 lost; showing an average proportion of one death in 11¾. This agrees remarkably with the success obtained in other countries.

These facts are derived from the reports of Admiral Mordvinow, then president of the Imperial Council, who affirms, that "Not a single death has occurred where Homœopathic treatment was resorted to in the incipient symptoms of the Cholera;" and that "it was remarked, that all the patients cured by Homœopathia, regained, in a very short time, their former health and strength; while those who survived other treatments, were left in a state of weakness which lasted several months, and but too often terminated in another disease which proved fatal."

The following is an extract from a letter which Admiral Mordvinow received from his daughter, Madame Lvoff, of the government of Saratow. It is dated August 6th, 1831.

"The dreadful Cholera broke out last month in our own village and its vicinity with the greatest fury. My husband was the first person attacked; but thanks to Homœopathia, was cured in a few days. From a desire to relieve the sufferings of humanity, he visited all the places in the neighborhood, where-ever the disease raged the most; administered the remedies; instructed the priests and the elders in the use of them; and was whole weeks thus employed, while I remained at home occupied with the preparation of Homœopathic powders. Four hundred Cholera patients, saved and restored to perfect health, was the gratifying reward of his zeal, and the triumphant result of Homœopathic doses liberally distributed to all who applied for them. We are all now so well convinced of the miraculous power of this system, that we cannot sufficiently deplore the ignorance that *cannot*, and still more the obstinate prejudice that *will not* invoke its aid, and thereby rescue relatives and friends from certain death. The Asiatic Cholera, preceded by terror, ushered in by danger, and followed by desolation, comes now, remains, and departs a harmless thing. Its cure is in reality easier than that of a fever. Multiplied experiments, and consequent confidence in Homœopathic treatment, have divested it of all its appalling attributes, by subjugating it entirely to the skill of man. We had fifty patients in our own village, and not *one* of them *died.* On the estate of my sister-in law, there were likewise a good many *cases,* but no *deaths.* There is also an abundance of reason to believe, that the fatal termination of the disease, wherever it occurred, was occasioned altogether by neglect, want of necessary precaution, or deviation from the rules of regimen prescribed by Homœopathia. All the sick who took medicine in strict conformity to the rules, were *saved,* although some of them were already in the state of collapse, which apparently precluded all hope. In this last stage there were not a few with their teeth clenched so fast that it was necessary to force them open for the purpose of introducing the medicine; and yet, on the very day following, they were relieved and convalescent! My good husband, from the constant intercourse with the sick, took the infection several times, but in every instance was restored by a few Homœopathic globules. In short, we consider ourselves perfectly safe from this dreaded scourge, whatever may be its potency and virulence. The repeated numerous trials have more than satisfied us, that in the presence of Homœopathia, with its five remedies only, the Asiatic Cholera is not a mortal disease, and still less so when encountered at it commencement."*

To the statistics above given, in relation to the first invasion of this disease, I need not add a word of comment, to show the immense superiority of the Homœopathic treatment. Such a uniformity in the results in so many places, and with such a number of patients, must speak convincingly to every intelligent and unprejudiced mind.

EPIDEMIC OF 1848—1849.

The Cholera which prevailed in England in 1848–1849, and in New-York in 1849, was equally severe with that of 1831–32. As the amount of homœopathic as compared with allopathic practice, in Great Britain and the United States, even during this last epidemic, was small, the character of the average results depended mainly upon that of the old system, as it did in the former epidemic invasions of the same malady.

Let us look at some of these results.

In an article, written in Liverpool, dated Feb. 24th, 1849, and relating to the official returns made to the government, respecting the number of cases, deaths and cures in Great Britain, from the com-

* "Homœopathia Revealed," by the Hon. Alexis Eustaphieve. Mr. Eustaphieve has a copy of the original documents. I find in the "Bibliothèque Homœopathique," the same extract, with a very few slight verbal discrepancies.

mencement of the epidemic, it is stated, that the Cholera returns have now swelled to cases 12,485.

Deaths	5,546
Recoveries	3,788
Remaining under treatment, or result not stated	3,164

Thus more than one-third had died, and more than two-thirds had not yet recovered.

The new system afforded much better results than this, even in practice among the poor. For example, at the Liverpool Homœopathic Dispensary, there were between July 25th, and Sept. 15th, 1849,

Cases of Cholera	162
Cures	119
Deaths	43
Per centage of deaths to cases .	26½

Let us next look at one or two results on the Atlantic and at our Quarantine.

The first seven cases which occurred on board the packet ship New-York, in Dec. 1848, died under calomel treatment. The ship arrived at the Quarantine at Staten-Island, near New-York, on the 2d of December, and landed the remaining eleven or twelve patients, who had survived longer under a comparatively inert treatment. From the statement of the captain, and the daily published reports of the health-officer, from Dec. 5th to Jan. 4th—when reports ceased to be published—it appears that in the ship before her arrival, and in the hospitals at the Quarantine since, there had occurred about ninety-six cases and fifty-two deaths, from Cholera. The cases at the Quarantine were under the care of the health-officer himself, a skilful allopathic physician, who, having the population of the buildings under his supervision, had an opportunity of instructing them in regard to premonitory symptoms, and it is to be presumed, of treating them in an early stage. Yet more than one-half died, under calomel and other allopathic treatment.

There is no instance on record, of such mortality among the same number of persons under homœopathic treatment, for Cholera, or for *any acute disease, whatever*, in any part of the world.

Again, on February 13th, 1849, Cholera broke out on board the ship Liverpool, bound to this port. Symptoms—Cramps, vomiting and purging. Attacks 50, deaths 40.

In the Cholera of 1849, the Board of Health of the City of New-York, required of the physicians of this city, a daily report of the cases and deaths occurring in their private practice. The results were published daily by their authority, during the greater part of the epidemic. But as the total results are not published in the formal and final report of the Board, we have no data for determining the average degree of success which attended the treatment in private practice.

I am, however, able to arrive at an approximate estimate, by means of such of their daily reports as

I was able to find in the daily newspapers, and to copy from them, in the months of June and July. My record extends from June 4th to July 31st inclusive, with the exception of six days, in which the numbers, if published, were not found.

As thus estimated, the following are the results of fifty-two days' private practice, chiefly allopathic, in this city.

Number of cases,	2,631.
Number of deaths,	915.
Per centage of deaths,	34.78,

i. e., about thirty-five out of a hundred cases died.

Thus according to these reports, about one-third of the cases in private practice were fatal. The approximation of this result to those generally obtained in private practice at other times, and in different parts of the world, affords evidence of the general truthfulness of the reports of results, to the same extent that cases were reported.

That approximation, and the fact that the deaths from Cholera in the list kept by the Board, were fewer than those in the report of the City Inspector, render it highly probable, that those physicians who for the whole or a portion of the season, neglected to report cases, did at least as generally neglect to report results; and as delinquency in the performance of these duties to the public and to science, cannot justify a presumption of peculiar fidelity, intelligence and skill, in the treatment of their patients, it is by no means probable that the addition of their reports, if complete, would have given to the general report of the Board of Health, a more favorable complexion.

The number of cures in private practice was not published.

The Board of Health required of the Resident Physician a report on the history of the epidemic of 1849 in this city. In this official report it is stated, that the number of persons admitted into the five hospitals was 1901.

Deaths,	1,021.
Cures,	880.
Per centage of cures,	46.29.
Per centage of deaths,	53.71.

It thus appears, that more than half of those admitted into the allopathic hospitals died.

The city authorities, by the advice of allopathic physicians, refused the application of the friends of Homœopathy, for the establishment of a Cholera hospital, in which those who chose might receive homœopathic treatment. Consequently, it is impossible to give any relative hospital statistics for this city. Whether this was the object aimed at by those who instigated the refusal of this reasonable demand, I will not presume to decide.* Neither will I affirm that the dread of an unfavorable comparison, had an influence in the suppression of the publication of the reported results in private practice; although no one

* For an examination of the reasons urged by the Medical Counsel, vide appendix to Joslin's "Principles of Homœopathy."

has denied that the reports of physicians were as reliable in 1849 as in 1832, when the total results were considered fit for publication. But the young giant was then an infant, and by no means so formidable here, as to deter public functionaries from the discharge of their official duties.

In order to obtain as authentic and official statistics of the reformed medical treatment, as was practicable under those circumstances, the Homœopathic Society of New-York, early in the epidemic, publicly requested the homœopathic physicians of New-York and Brooklyn, to report to them, through their Secretary, such cases of Cholera as they had reported to the Mayor, Board of Health, or Resident Physician, and also the results as so reported.

This plan of confining the Society reports to cases and deaths reported to the city authorities, who were under the influence of a rival school, jealous and vigilant, and possessed, by means of these reports, of the names and residences of the patients, within twenty-four hours of the occurrence of the case or death, affords to our opponents sufficient security, that the society reports would not be too favorable to the reputation of our system. This plan also gives to the statistics a semi-official character.

Twenty-two physicians, (twenty-one of them residing in New-York proper,) complied with the request of the Society, and the results were published weekly, from July 12th, by its Secretary, B. F. Bowers, M. D.

These reports embrace the cases which occurred in their practice, from the commencement to the termination of the epidemic.

To those who are acquainted with these physicians, their names are a sufficient guarantee for the truthfulness of their reports.

I give them as they stand on the Secretary's list, in the order of the commencement of the reports to him. They are: Drs. Bayard, Stewart, Joslin, Cator, Bowers, Bolles, Ball, Taylor, Wright, Kinsley, Freeman, Allen, Baldwin, Kirby, Quin, Moffat, Stearns, Hallock, Wilsey, Denison, Sherrill, and McVickar.

The following table exhibits the results of reports to the Society, in the periods there stated, said reports referring respectively to previous ones made to the municipal authorities.

	Cases.	Deaths.
In one week, in 1849, previously to July 12,	59	8
" " from July 12 to 19,	23	4
" " " " 19 to 26,	37	2
" " " " 26 to Aug. 2,	43	9
" " " Aug. 2 to 9,	26	5
" " " " 9 to 16,	47	5
" " " " 16 to 13,	42	6
" " " " 23 to 30,	13	2
" " " " 30 to Sept. 6,	11	3
" " " Sept. 6 to 13,	7	2
" " " " 13 to 20,	3	1

	Cases.	Deaths.
In one week, from Sept. 20 to 27,	1	1
Reports postponed,*	37	5
Case reported October 9th,	1	0
Total,	350	53

Per centage of deaths $15\frac{1}{7}$.

It appears from this, that the mortality in private homœopathic practice was about fifteen per cent.; whilst the mortality in the average private practice of the city, for the time embraced in our records, was about thirty-five per cent.

The results would afford a comparison still more favorable for Homœopathy, if we excluded from the average results in the city, that portion which was reported by homœopathic physicians. If the Board of Health had reported the total number of cases and deaths in private practice, and if all the homœopathic physicians had made a similar report in regard to their practice, we should have had the requisite data for a more satisfactory solution of the problem of the relative merits of the two systems. It is evident from the advantage which the general results derived from the more favorable homœopathic results incorporated in them, that had it been in our power to obtain a complete report, it would have exhibited results still more favorable to the reputation of the new method.

But were it possible to effect this separation, and

* Reported to the Board of Health some time previously to the 20th and before the 27th, to the Secretary.

institute a comparison between the reports of the new and those of the old school, the tables would, even then, be far from exhibiting the full superiority of the actual curative results of the new method.

Because—First; the want of a homœopathic hospital threw a greater number of desperate cases into the private practice of homœopathic physicians. Secondly; a greater number of desperate cases were transferred from other physicians to them, than from them to others. Thirdly; fewer homœopathic cholera patients died from other diseases, after reaction. Fourthly; many of them were cured by domestic camphor treatment, and consequently were not reported.

I will consider some of these points more particularly.

Those who have an opportunity of practising extensively during the whole of a severe cholera epidemic, will see so many cases among the moral, sober, intelligent and wealthy, as to cease to consider the disease disgraceful or ungenteel—if he had previously indulged such a prejudice. There is much less difference between the rich and the poor, in their liability to an attack of this disease, than in their danger of dying by it. But fatal cases do occur in a much greater proportion among the latter.

The poor of our city having been, by the municipal government, denied the advantage of a homœopathic hospital, many of them, who preferred the treatment of our physicians, had to be attended in such a state of want, and in localities so crowded and impure, that they would have been removed to a hospital, had one existed for our school. Our professional brethren of the other school were, in private practice, often relieved from such unpromising cases. I am of opinion, that nearly all the fatal cholera cases which it became the duty of the homœopathic physicians of this city to report, occurred either among the poor, or else among comparative strangers to the physician, and even to the practice. The latter were persons who applied to us for aid, after having exhausted their own resources, or those of their allopathic physician. In my own practice, no family which had employed me previously to the epidemic, or even previously to the occurrence of the case, lost any of its members by cholera. Yet fifty cases occurred among these my own proper families, and were all cured.

Some of our cases came under our care and were reported by us, after their condition had become desperate under allopathic practice; whilst comparatively few, and I have not heard that any, of our cases were transferred to the old school under similar circumstances.

A homœopathic cure is a cure in reality; an allopathic cure is often merely a transfer of disease to a different organ, or an exchange of one morbid action for another. The apparent cure of cholera by large doses, gave rise in numerous instances, to local congestions of vital organs, typhoid fevers, &c. There is little doubt that in private practice, the deaths in

5

these cases were in many instances, reported under the name applicable to the form which the disease last assumed, especially where the death occurred a long time after reaction had been established.

Now there is little chance for homœopathy to improve its cholera statistics by such occurrences. For these new forms of disease are extremely rare after homœopathic treatment. The cholera, once apparently cured by small doses, is really cured.

The Board of Health required no reports of cures; but I rendered them, in order that they might have data for testing the reality of the cures, and verifying the totality of my reports. In a report made to the President of the Board on the 7th of September, 1849, after giving the names of eight persons recently cured of cholera, (there were no new cases nor deaths to report) I added the following remarks: Of every case of cholera reported by me, I have reported the result. You will find, that the numbers of patients which I have reported as cured of cholera, and died of cholera, will, when added together, equal the number which I have reported as attacked with cholera.

Finally, great numbers who were attacked with Cholera, were cured immediately by their domestic attendants, with that use of Camphor which we had advised. In some of these instances, the physician was not called; in others, on arriving he found the patient so far recovered, that he could not report it as a case of Cholera then under his care.

If the influence of all these facts were duly estimated in the statistics, it would be found, that Homœopathy had not lost one-fourth as large a proportion of its cases as allopathy, and had cured nearly as great a proportion in this as in former epidemics.

As evidence of the extent of the domestic Camphor treatment in this city, so far as the influence of nearly all the principal homœopathic physicians could secure its adoption, and as affording also a model for circulars to the public in any place where Cholera prevails, I insert the following card, which those physicians published, and distributed as widely as possible among the families which they attended.

ADVICE TO THE PUBLIC IN RELATION TO CHOLERA.

NEW-YORK, June 2d, 1849.

The undersigned, Physicians of the city of New-York, believing that during the prevalence of Cholera, many lives are in danger of being sacrificed to improper modes of treatment, recommended in the newspapers, consider it their duty to warn the public of the danger of using the drugs generally recommended, and large doses of medicine of any kind. Since homœopathy has saved 91 out of 100 in thousands of cases of Cholera, we feel confident that it will cure almost every case, provided the physician is called immediately after the attack, and before any other treatment has been resorted to. But if any other medicine beside the appropriate homœopathic remedies are employed, or if several hours elapse, before the proper treatment is commenced, the cure will in many cases be impracticable by any treatment.

It is important that the community should be especially warned against the use of Laudanum and Opium in any form, as well as calomel and all the advertised specifics.

During the prevalence of Cholera, every person should immediately consult his physician for the slightest diarrhœa, (whether with or without pain,) avoiding Laudanum, and also cathartics even of the mildest kind. If medical advice cannot be obtained within an hour or two, the patient may take spirits of Camphor a few times, in a dose of one drop.

Every person attacked with such diarrhœa, vomiting, cramps, colic or other symptoms, as give an apprehension that actual Cholera has commenced, should take one drop of spirits of Camphor in sugared water, every five minutes, and nothing else, until relief is obtained, or the physician arrives.

Twelve drops of the Camphor, dropped in a table-spoonful of white sugar, may be dissolved in twelve table-spoonfuls of cold water, and one table-spoonful of this solution be given every five minutes. This, in most cases, will make an excellent foundation for the complete cure by the physician; but he should be immediately called, whatever may be the apparent amendment.

Spirits of Camphor should not be used in large doses as a curative, nor by persons in health, in any dose, with the expectation of preventing the disease; but we believe that appropriate homœopathic medicines are efficacious as preventives.

We have not here given any advice for the use of other medicines beside Camphor, believing it impracticable to point out the indications for each in a few words. Those who cannot consult a physician will find full directions in works written expressly on this subject.*

J. H. Allen, M.D.	B. F. Joslin, M.D.
A. S. Ball, M.D.	Hudson Kinsley, M.D.
S. B. Barlow, M.D.	S. R. Kirby, M.D.
Edward Bayard, M.D.	M. E. Lazarus, M.D.
J. Beakley, M.D.	John Aug. McVickar, M.D.
Clare W. Beames, M.D.	James M. Quin, M.D.
R. M. Bolles, M.D.	H. Sherrill, M.D.
B. F. Bowers, M.D.	Danl. E. Stearns, M.D.
J. Bowers, M.D.	W. Stewart, M.D.
H. Hull Cator, M.D.	J. Taylor, M.D.
Wm. Channing, M.D.	F. L. Wilsey, M.D.
Alfred Freeman, M.D.	Clark Wright, M.D.
Chas. J. Hempel, M.D.	

The cases of diarrhœa and other choleroid affections, treated by the homœopathic physicians of New-York during this epidemic, were probably eight or ten times as numerous as those which they re-

* The first edition of this book had been published in March. The advice in the above circular is, so far as it extends, in accordance with the book, and for this reason is, to that extent, a recommendation of it by the physicians signing the circular.

garded and reported as Cholera.* As those diarrhœas and other choleroid cases were all cured, the addition of their number to that of the Cholera cases, would reduce the per-centage of deaths to less than two. It would not however be fair to take advantage of such a combination, in estimating the relative success of the two systems. Candor requires the acknowledgment, that most allopathic physicians in our city probably agreed with us in not reporting cases of mere cholerine or other choleroid affections. Both schools reported only cases of developed Cholera.

In Cincinnati, Ohio, during the epidemic of 1849, the extent and success of the homœopathic treatment were remarkable.

Drs. Pulte and Ehrmann of that City used the one-drop doses of Camphor with almost universal success, early in the disease. In more advanced cases, they employed homœopathic attenuations, of Arsenicum, Carb.-v., Cuprum, Secale, Veratrum, &c.

They had cases of Cholera .	1,116
Deaths, only	35
Per-centage of deaths . . .	$3\frac{1}{7}$

This brilliant success, the saving of about 97 cases in a hundred, seems to have been attained in the use of Camphor which would be considered excessively small by the soi-disant regular physicians, and by other medicines in a state so dilute, that the doses would be regarded as inefficient or unre-

* If I may judge from Dr. Kinsley's records and my own.

liable by such of our school as confine their practice chiefly to mother tinctures extemporaneously diluted, and to the first attenuation. Dr. Pulte, in those instances in which, in his "Domestic Physician" since published, he states the particular attenuations to be given in Cholera, generally recommends high dilutions; in only one instance (that of Prussic-acid), the second, in one (that of Veratrum), the 12th; whilst of Arsenicum, Carbo-veg., Cuprum and Secale, he recommends no other than the 30th dilution. Such it may be presumed was his practice; and I was informed at that time, that Drs. Pulte and Ehrmann used high dilutions in that epidemic.

In addition to these cases of Cholera, they treated 1,350 cases of cholerine or diarrhœa, all of which, as well as the dysenteries, were cured. The success of the homœopathic treatment in dysentery, provided the medicines are sufficiently attenuated, is every where remarkable.

In the large number of cholera cases, as compared with diarrhœas, the epidemic in Cincinnati might appear, from the above account to have been remarkably different from that in New-York, the same year; also from that in Liverpool, where, according to Dr. Drysdale's article in the British Journal, the number of cases of cholerine, diarrhœa and dysentery, treated at the Liverpool Homœopathic Dispensary that year, amounted to upwards of 1,000 whilst the number of cases of Cholera, treated by the physicians of the dispensary was 175.

Some cholera statistics are given by Dr. Russell of Edinburgh and Dr. Drysdale of Liverpool, in two elaborate and ably-written articles in the British Journal of Homœopathy, Vol. 7th and 8th, from the last of which a part of the preceding information has been obtained. They describe many cases. The dilutions ranged from the first to the sixth.

At the Liverpool Homœopathic Dispensary, in 1849, among patients in indigent circumstances, and consequently, when attacked, more liable than others to die of Cholera, the per-centage of deaths was $25\frac{71}{100}$.

In the same city for three months, in the practice of physicians mainly allopathic, the per-centage was 46.

At the Edinburgh Homœopathic Dispensary, there were, from the 8th of October to the 6th of December, 1848:

Cases of Cholera	173
Recoveries	124
Deaths	48
Under treatment at the time of the report	1
Per-centage of deaths	$27\frac{32}{43}$.

This being, like that reported at Liverpool, dispensary practice, and consequently among the poor, the results should be compared with something intermediate between allopathic hospital and private practice, to show the relative success of the two systems.

In the cases included in the statistics given in this book, the average New-York doses, were smaller than those of Edinburgh and Liverpool; and larger than those of Cincinnati in the same year, and those of continental Europe in the first epidemic. The results afford some evidence in favor of the higher dilutions, in all these groups of cases as compared with each other. The same conclusion in favor of the higher potencies may be drawn from the relative success of Drs. Meyerhœfer and Fleischmann, at the Hospital of the Sisters of Charity in Vienna, during the first two epidemics.

As there may be other circumstances beside the treatment, that modify the results, we should attach no great importance to the evidence afforded by two such classes of facts, as compared merely with each other; but with an increase in the number of corroborative classes, the probability increases in a ratio vastly higher than that in which the number increases. The above coincidences appear to me sufficiently numerous to merit serious consideration.

From considerations of delicacy, I have refrained from giving the average results in the practice of individual physicians, either as bearing upon the relative success of the two schools, or that of the different shades of our own.

Had the materials been accessible, it would have been gratifying to publish a more comprehensive statement of the results of the homœopathic and allopathic methods of practice in the epidemic of 1849. Such numerical statements as I have met with have been introduced into this book, provided they were well authenticated, and referred to numbers sufficiently large to afford a probable approximation to the general average of the results of either method in any considerable population. They have been impartially selected on the principles above stated, and not with any reference to their comparative bearing upon the reputation of our system. The results (so far as known) under homœopathic treatment in Edinburgh, Liverpool, New-York and Cincinnati, were:

Cases of Cholera	1813
Deaths from Cholera	181
Per-centage of deaths . . .	$9\frac{98}{100}$

i. e. the mortality was nearly ten per-cent.

The probability that this is a near approximation to the general average for our school, is increased by combining the above numbers with others referring to a previous epidemic in other places. Thus, under the homœopathic treatment, in Russia and Austria, and at Berlin and Paris, in 1831 and 1832, in Edinburgh in 1848, and in Liverpool, New-York and Cincinnati in 1849, there were, so far as the statistics could be collected:

Cases of Cholera	4,830
Deaths from Cholera	445
Per-centage of deaths $9\frac{1}{4}$, or exactly	$9\frac{21}{100}$.

That is, on an average, under the system of Hahnemann about 91 out of a hundred attacked with this terrible malady have been saved.

Allopathy loses about four times as large a proportion of its Cholera cases; or three times as many in practice exclusively private.

Avoiding any attempt to make out a case by special pleading, I have here summed up the numbers as they are found without modification.

This is a subject on which the simple expression of the naked mathematical truth, may to many seem like satire and self-laudation. Such a view would do injustice to the spirit in which these estimates have been undertaken, and their inevitable conclusions exhibited. Whilst we lament the impotence of our art in many cases of complete collapse, and an average mortality in developed cases in general, exceeding that in many other maladies, it is proper to search for the exact truth in relation to the absolute and relative success of the two methods, and to state it for the confirmation and consolation of new proselytes, and the persuasion of sceptics and opponents.

Grateful to the Author of all good for the knowledge of this beneficient system, we are desirous that others should appreciate and enjoy its advantages; but we claim no innate superiority for ourselves, nor any perfection for the details of our practice. The law of Hahnemann is an immutable verity; but we hope for ampler materials, as the media of its application. We desire that the powerful intellects which are now wasted in the toils of a field comparatively barren, should be directed to a science whose cultivation is sure to be rewarded with new and practical truth. The distinctive appellations for the two principal sects, now existing in the medical world, are applied to them for the sake of precision, not the one as boastful, the other contemptuous. They are both equally expressive and respectful; but we hope for a distant future, when the universal adoption of our system shall render such distinctions unnecessary and obsolete, and the terms allopathist and homœopathist be known only in history.

In giving the statistics which I have been able to collect for the epidemic of 1849, I have not alluded to informal accounts, unaccompanied by exact numerical statements; though these more vague accounts of the treatment in the cities of Europe and America, are every where favorable to our system, from Petersburgh and Riga in the North-East, to St. Louis and New-Orleans in the South-West.

I shall conclude this chapter with an item of recent news, illustrating the ravages of the pestilence at the commencement of the present year, the self-sacrificing zeal with which a Christian minister could peril his health, liberty and life, when sustained by confidence in homœopathic truth, and a sense of duty to suffering humanity.

CHOLERA IN 1854.

During the past winter, the Cholera, as is usual at that season, has been almost exclusively confined to warm climates. We have accounts of its ravages in some of the West India islands, and in some portions of Central America, but not many facts in relation to its treatment or statistics.

The following is an interesting extract from a letter from Rev. Frederick Crowe, a Baptist Missionary in Balize, Honduras, dated 2d February, 1854, directed to Mr. C. T. Hurlbut, a homœopathic pharmaceutist of New-York. After ordering for a friend a supply of medicines, and the most necessary homœopathic books, he adds:

"Any tracts on the first principles of homœopathy, that you can add, would be of use here, as the system has been hitherto unknown, save by vague report.

"My arrival here with the supply I had of you was timely. Three weeks ago the Cholera broke out; and it has been raging ever since, so that ten or twelve have died daily, in a population of 8,000. One day twenty-six died. We hear reports of much greater mortality in the surrounding country.

"I felt it my duty to put by every other occupation and attend exclusively to the sick; using the homœopathic treatment of course. This drew down the opposition of the medical men, the Board of Health and I regret to add, of the ministers of religion, of all the other denominations. I was threatened with a trial for my life on the first case of death under my treatment. I felt it my duty to proceed, and bear any penalty that might follow; and I soon found that public opinion protected me from any overt acts on the part of the enemies of the system.

"I printed the directions of which I enclose you a copy, both in English and Spanish, and being ably seconded by Mr. Henderson, and more or less assisted by several of our native teachers, the homœopathic treatment soon became general, and the usual practice almost exceptional.

"I believe that hundreds have been preserved by the means we used—as the Camphorated Spirits of Wine may now be found in almost every house in the settlement, and it is resorted to at once by the poor people on the first appearance of the terrible malady. Many cases I have superintended myself, laboring night and day, as far as my strength would permit; and in order to make that go further, I hired a horse, and looked for all the world like the regular practitioners—which I fear has provoked them still more.

"My success has been highly encouraging. Out of scores of cases, for I soon lost count, only five or six have died while I attended them; and several of them were tampered with by the Allopathists or by the misguided zeal of friends, either previously to, or during my treatment, and others were far gone before I was called in.

"I may yet be called to suffer for what I have done, as I am not licensed, (to kill or cure,) but I am prepared for the worst; and am satisfied that I have only done my duty. The poor people are grateful, and a Homœopathic doctor would have no difficulty in getting into good general practice here, on the strength of the present excitement.

"In one of the hospitals improvised for the occasion, not a single patient recovered. But three patients left it in a panic before they were either killed or cured. It now goes by the name of the slaughter house. The method pursued by our opponents is terrific.—Draughts of Cayenne pepper, or pills of the same, large doses of ammonia, confection of opium and prepared chalk, with rubbings of turpentine, and both frictions with, and plentiful draughts of raw brandy, upon the Cayenne, &c.—These are their principal agents. As you may suppose, few could stand such treatment, and the Cholera too. Either one alone, a good, strong constitution might grapple with and recover.

"I intend to write to Dr. Joslin, whose book on Cholera has been of much use to me—and to the journal also—but hitherto I have had no time. You are at liberty to publish any part of this."

CHAPTER IV.

EARLY TREATMENT,

DOMESTIC AND PROFESSIONAL,

INCLUDING THAT OF THE PREMONITORY SYMPTOMS, AND OF THE DISEASE AT ITS ONSET, WITH DIRECTIONS FOR THE GENERAL MANAGEMENT.

DOMESTIC AND PROFESSIONAL TREATMENT OF PREMONITORY SYMPTOMS, AND THE SLIGHTER ATTACKS.

During the prevalence of Cholera in any locality, every person should consult his physician for such slight symptoms as often precede Cholera. On such application to the physician, if a homœopathist, the disease may almost always be warded off, or, if commencing in a slight form, immediately cured, and prevented from advancing into the form of Cholera proper. The most usual premonitory symptom is a fœcal diarrhœa, often so slight that it would excite no apprehension in ordinary times. Or the evacuations may be rather copious, or in moderate quantity and milky, no other symptoms being present. In any of these forms, diarrhœa in the epidemic is called Cholerine. It will be again referred to as the first stage of the first variety of Cholera; yet the importance of an early attention to it is so great, that at the expense of some repetition, a familiar account of its symptoms and first treatment are given in this place, for the convenience of such families as may use this book, and physicians hitherto unacquainted with this practice.

Where there is diarrhœa without any special indication for any particular remedy, give one drop of spirits of *Camphor*, on a lump of sugar or in sugared water. Give another drop after one hour,—or earlier, if the diarrhœa returns—and let it be followed by three doses of the 3d attenuation of Camphor, at intervals of an hour, or after each evacuation, if it occurs sooner; after this, if the diarrhœa continues, *Phosphorus* ^{30}; if the tongue sticks a little to the finger when applied to it, give *Phosphoric*-acid; if it has a yellowish coat, and there is colic or dizziness, give Veratrum ^{30}. Whichever medicine is given, it may be repeated after each evacuation, if it is large, or after every two, if they are small.

For other symptoms consult the succeeding chapters, including the Repertories, Chapters X and XI.*

The *Camphor* may also be used for a short time, with advantage for most *other symptoms;* but if this is domestic treatment, there should be no unnecessary delay in consulting a Homœopathic physician;

* The principal divisions of the Repertories, are in the order in which it would be most natural to examine (from above downwards) those different parts of the body to which the symptoms belong; whilst the subordinate arrangement, that of the different parts of each section of the repertory, is alphabetical.

as the disease may reach a dangerous height before the appropriate remedy is employed.

In giving pellets of any medicine, in the dry state, a good general rule is: Put two or three pellets in a small powder of pure sugar or sugar of milk, fold the paper, then mash the pellets, then open the paper, and mix them by moving the paper without touching the powder. Then with the paper bent at an angle, place its edges in contact with the upper lip or teeth, let the powder slide on the tongue without touching it with the paper. The patient should hold his head back, his mouth open, and his tongue out, and allow the powder to dissolve on the tongue before swallowing it.

Where a number of doses of any one medicine are to be given in succession, it is more convenient and equally effectual to dissolve five or six pellets in a gill of water, and give one, two or three teaspoonfuls—according to the patient's age—at a dose. This may be considered as applying to any case, in this or or any other stage.

DOMESTIC AND PROFESSIONAL TREATMENT AT THE COMMENCEMENT OF CHOLERA IN ALL ITS FORMS.

When there is a decided attack of Cholera, we resort for the first hour, or a longer or shorter time according to circumstances, to a treatment for which, as well as for all the most successful modes of preventing and curing this disease, the world is indebted to Hahnemann.

Whatever may be the form of the attack, give one drop of the tincture of Camphor, dropped on a lump of sugar, and then dissolved in a tablespoonful of cold water. Repeat this every five minutes, until there is a decided mitigation of the symptoms. This will usually be after five or six doses. One sign of its good effect is perspiration. In proportion as the symptoms yield, let the doses be at longer intervals, as an hour, two hours, twelve and even twenty-four hours. For these later doses, the third attenuation would probably be preferable. If the disease is taken in time, ten or twelve doses of the tincture are ordinarily sufficient. If the stomach will not retain the Camphor, even in ice-water, then give, before and after it, a bit of ice as large as a filbert; or reduce the dose to one-quarter of a drop, if necessary. In order to commence immediately, the first dose may be a drop on a lump of sugar; but as soon as there is time, dissolve it as hereafter directed.

The patient should continue in bed and be covered, for many hours, as exertion and check of the perspiration excited by the Camphor, would both at first tend to prevent improvement, and afterwards to occasion relapse, even after the cure had considerably advanced.

In the preparation of this spirits of Camphor, Hahnemann recommended the proportion of one oz. of solid Camphor (the gum as it is called) to twelve of alcohol. Dr. Quin used the proportion of one to six. The usual tincture of the shops is suitable. The method which is most convenient and useful, and one which I have employed in many cases of severe Cholera, is to put twelve drops of camphorated spirits in a tablespoonful of sugar, and dissolve it in twelve tablespoonfuls of cold water in a tumbler, and give a tablespoonful of this mixture every five minutes till relief is obtained. Where there is great difficulty in retaining fluids on the stomach, let the medicine be so dissolved that a teaspoonful shall be a dose. If the water were not rendered viscid by sugar, much of the Camphor would rise to the surface, and if the spirits were dropped into water first, the Camphor would be precipitated at the surface.

Families should be provided with the Camphor, and in case of attack administer it immediately before the arrival of the physician, who will judge whether it is to be continued. In some cases of severe spasms, it might perhaps be admissible to give the Camphor every third minute, till there was some mitigation. But the advantages of the Camphor treatment cannot be secured by Allopathic doses, whether at short or long intervals. In the former case, the disease would be aggravated; and in the latter case, the medicinal action would become exhausted: in both cases, the stomach would be irritated. If one ignorantly attempts to correct the last effect by combining Opium or Laudanum with the Camphor, he, in a great measure, destroys the efficacy of the latter, besides doing direct and positive injury by the opiate.

There is abundant testimony to the efficacy of the pure Camphor treatment (by small doses) from all parts of Europe.

Hahnemann states, that at Berlin and Magdeburg alone, thousands of families having followed his instructions respecting the treatment by Camphor, restored those of their members who were attacked by the epidemic—restored them often in less than a quarter of an hour. This method was said to be employed with certainty of success in the first hour; with probability in the following hours. Now, it sometimes fails, oftener among children. I recommend the trial of pellets, and not lower than Camph.^{1}, even for adults. Probably the Camph.$^{\circ}$ will soon be less used.

Hahnemann at first advised the external, in connexion with the internal, use of Camphor, but subsequently found it unnecessary. Indeed it not only is useless, but fills the room with effluvia which interfere with subsequent treatment.

But as it is often difficult to persuade the friends of the patient to wait for the action of the remedy, they may be allowed to rub with a flannel, either dry, or moistened with alcohol, or—what is better—with their dry hands. They may also be allowed to place a warm brick at the feet of the patient—if they are cold—although it is of no positive use.

Though Camphor has not, on the whole, lost any reputation in the epidemic of 1849, yet I have been informed of several instances of its failure, even when given under the above favorable circumstances, and apparently in cases to which it was appropriate —and have seen it and other remedies fail, where Laudanum had been previously given, and several hours had elapsed, before the homœopathic physician was called.

From the general utility of the early employment of Camphor, it is not to be inferred that the homœopathic physician will usually commence with it, where the family, instructed in its use, has given many doses of it previously to his arrival. His course will be determined by a consideration of the totality of the symptoms.

Though the Camphor should produce immediate relief, it is not to be relied on for a permanent cure, where one or more other medicines are subsequently indicated by the symptoms—as will often be the case. After such improvement, the patient will be safe with other appropriate treatment, but not always without it.

Camphor is a remedy which is imperfectly proved, as to the symptoms which it is capable of producing in the attenuated, and even in the crude state; and our school has more experience of its use in cholera in the former than in the latter condition. These are reasons for employing it in a form less attenuated than that adopted for other medicines. Another reason is, that the poison of cholera is probably of animalcular origin, and Camphor neutralizes the poison of many insects.*

These considerations justify the use of drop doses of Camphor; and the use of such doses, so far as the object is to act directly on a *poison in* the body, affords no evidence of our inconsistency, or lack of confidence in infinitissimal doses, when we employ them to act *directly on the human organism*, and restore its healthy action. Those who are not satisfied with this brief explanation, or desire a more extensive examination of the subject of antidotes, and the use of mechanical and chemical means and large doses, in

* The prevalent opinion, that Camphor is a medicine which does not bear much attenuation, has not been established by experiments. Of the high attenuation, I know of no other proving than the following:

In 1849, on Tuesday evening, Feb. 22d, at twenty minutes of ten, I took a few dry pellets of Bœnnenghausen's Camphor $_{200}$, and administered the same dose to Dr. H. H. Cator and Mr. (now Dr.) Brown. In twelve minutes I had cold perspiration, especially on the forehead and chest. The same symptom was simultaneously experienced by the two other provers. In the epidemic of the following summer, Dr. B. F. Bowers employed Camph. ^{200} with success in many cholera cases, and was as well satisfied of the reality of its curative action, as of that of any other remedy. He frequently took it himself when he experienced any premonitory symptoms, but never in any other form than the 200th, during the epidemic. In the present month, April, 1854, I have administered Camph. $_{30}$, with immediate and complete success, for cholera diarrhœa with milky discharges. The 30th and lower potencies of Camphor have been employed successfully by Drs. Barlow, Bayard and Kirby.

connection with homœopathic treatment, are referred to my volume on "Principles."*

In conclusion I must add, that the large doses of Camphor, used in popular and allopathic practice, dangerously oppress the stomach and brain, and frustrate the cure.

DIRECTIONS FOR THE GENERAL MANAGEMENT OF A CHOLERA PATIENT.

1. Apply no camphor externally, and use no external applications of any kind.

2. Give no drinks but cold water, unless the patient prefers warm toast water, which is the case in but very few instances.

3. Ice water may be taken as frequently as the patient desires it. It is useful for extreme thirst, cramps, colic, vomiting and cold skin.

4. The food should consist of mutton or chicken broth, with no seasoning except a moderate quantity of salt. Beef broth will answer. Oyster soup is not allowed. Great care should be used in regard to diet during convalescence.

5. The patient should lie in bed, with comfortable coverings.

6. If the weather is cool, there should be a good fire, which will allow the windows to be kept open for ventilation.

---

* Vide, "Principles of Homœopathy," Lecture 3d.

7. The patient should not, however, be exposed to cold air. If compelled to rise, he should be covered, and the windows closed.

8. He should rise no oftener, and move no more, than necessary; as motion is hurtful. He should, if practicable, be provided with a bed-pan, instead of being compelled to rise.

9. No glass or spoon which has been used for one medicine, should be used for another, until it has been rinsed with clean hot water, (without soap,) then, whilst hot, wiped dry with a clean towel, and allowed to stand till cool, and thus become more perfectly dried by its own heat. Or when convenient, it should be washed with hot water, and wiped, then heated near a fire, and again allowed to cool before being used for another medicine.

CHAPTER VII.

SYMPTOMS AND TREATMENT OF THE VARIETIES OF CHOLERA.

LAW OF CURE, AND REPETITION AND MAGNITUDE OF DOSES.

The skilful Homœopathic physician does not neglect the teachings of clinical experience; but he relies mainly on the law, that any disease, in its curable stage, can be cured by a medicine which is capable of producing a sufficiently large group of symptoms similar to those which the disease itself presents.* Judgment is required in regard to the relative importance of symptoms; but it is important to consult repertories and materia medicas with regard to a great number of the symptoms of a case, and to combine as many as possible, and thus eliminate the false remedies and arrive at the true remedy for the whole group, and consequently for the disease of which that group is the index or exponent. The popular error, that a knowledge of the name, essential nature and principal seat of the disease, is pre-requisite to a successful treatment of it, is founded upon the blind nature of allopathic therapeutics. Allopathy has no guide but the name, the supposed nature and the supposed seat of the malady: and if any one who has received some homœopathic light, allows himself to be still led by the blind, he will fall into the same ditch.

The usual intervals between the doses of attenuated medicines for the more severe varieties of Cholera are, half an hour, one hour, and an hour and a half, according to the violence of the disease. In some violent cases, the medicine may be repeated in fifteen minutes. But we are not to suppose that the good effect is ordinarily increased by this greater frequency,

* For proofs of the truth and advantages of this law, see my "Principles of Homœopathy," Lecture IV.

or that too frequent a repetition is harmless. Again, we are not to suppose, that the operation of an attenuated medicine will be frustrated by the occurrence of vomiting at the end of several minutes after it has been swallowed. It is not like a crude drug. Some portion of it has already gone to every part of the body; and the portions which have entered the circulation have nearly as much power as the whole dose.

Vomiting after such an interval does not render a repetition of the dose necessary. Neither are we to suppose that the dose requires to be repeated on account of the patient's having taken food or drink which is slightly medicinal or antidotal. It is not probable that the action of an attenuated medicine can be entirely frustrated by antidotes taken in the crude form. The attenuations have peculiar power. Every experienced and observant homœopathic physician knows, that less than a billionth part of a grain of common salt, will manifest its specific effects in an individual who is taking many grains of crude salt at every meal. The rule of three fails to explain the effect of such an infinitesimal increase in the quantity. The inference is inevitable, that the homœopathic process has developed immense power.* The existence of great curative power in the homœopathic attenuations is manifested by their effects on cholera.

* For other proofs of this, see a more extensive examination of the "power of small doses," in the second lecture of the volume, referred to in the preceding note.

The proper attenuations for the respective medicines are stated in the Introduction. They are, in most of them, the 12th or 30th. They may be given dry, in loaf sugar or sugar of milk, or in solution in iced water. Iced water is itself a remedy, and it may be given to the patient in most cases. In regard to the repetition of attenuated medicines, a rule applicable to all cases of Cholera is—discontinue the administration of medicine as soon as there is amendment, and as long as this is progressive.

In regard to dose and mode of administration, consult Chapter VI.

In the case of camphor, as compared with other medicines, the dose is large and the repetitions frequent; for it is unlike all other medicines in not requiring attenuation, and in being exceedingly transient in its action. Hahnemann directed one drop of the tincture every five minutes; the tincture being made by dissolving one oz. of camphor in twelve of alcohol. Dr. Quin happened to use, in his own case, two-drop doses of the tincture, made in the proportion of one to six, and finding it to succeed, used it for others. Hartmann recommends the proportion of one to twenty, and the dose one or two drops, every two or five minutes. The tincture directed by the allopathic pharmacopæias and found in the drugstores, is generally one to eight, sometimes one to sixteen. There is probably no better rule, than to dissolve one oz. of camphor in ten oz. (i. e. 2½ gills) of alcohol.* The ordinary dose will be one drop every five minutes. In some cases, the dose may be increased to two drops, or the intervals reduced to two or three minutes. Give the tincture in sugared water, iced or at least cold. As camphor is one of the most powerful and general antidotes to other medicines, the patient must not take these from any glass or spoon which has contained it, nor must the odor of it be in the room after he commences other medicines.

The forms described in this Chapter are those which the Cholera most frequently presents. Some of them are occasionally combined. The Homœopathic physician will know how to adapt his treatment to the different shades and combinations of these varieties.† He will apply the Materia Medica, and the law similia similibus curantur. The accompanying Repertories will aid in the selection of the remedies.

SYMPTOMS OF THE FIRST VARIETY, CHOLERA DIARRHŒICA INTESTINAL, OR DIARRHŒIC CHOLERA.

This is the form in which *diarrhœa* is a prominent symptom. At first there is a simple diarrhœa; las-

---

* This is the strength of the tincture which the publisher (Wm. Radde) will sell with this book.

† The term varieties, is not used in this book to denote unusual forms of this disease, but the more usual forms of the Cholera considered as itself a species.

situde in the legs ; rumblings ; tongue moist, clean or a little coated ; sometimes it is pasty, or gluey, so as to adhere to the finger when applied to it. The evacuations, at first composed of digested food or feculent matters, shortly become yellowish brown or watery: after a few hours or a few days, they have the appearance of barley-water, rice-water, or of whey with little flocks of soap distributed through it, or of milk-porridge mixed with water. The whiteness appears to depend on minute flocculi of whitish mucus, with some larger lumps of the same, sometimes as large as a pepper-corn and of a yellowish-white color. Each stool is preceded by great noise and movements in the intestines. The noise is sometimes like the rumbling of gas, at others like that of a running liquid. There is a livid circle around the eyes, or dark color of the whole face, coldness of the hands or tongue, prostration of muscular strength, and feebleness of pulse; sometimes nausea or cramps. Some vomiting may take place, after the diarrhœa has continued a considerable time without appropriate treatment.

If this form of Cholera, although it should amount only to a slight cholerine, is mistaken for an ordinary diarrhœa and improperly treated, there is great danger of its suddenly assuming a much graver form: vomiting and violent spasms may set in, and collapse and death close the scene. This alarming revolution in the disease may occur when the evacuations have not caused much debility or interfered with the usual avocations. In Europe and America, this diarrhœic form is the most frequent, especially in places and times in which Cholera does not rage in its greatest intensity. The most perfect and severe forms give no such warning, even in Europe and America.

In one sense, the premonitory diarrhœa is a part of the diarrhœic variety of Cholera. If a line can be drawn between them, it is probably where the discharges change from the fœcal to the liquid character. The treatment is similar.

TREATMENT OF DIARRHŒIC CHOLERA.*

If *Camphor* does not soon give relief, we are to resort to other medicines, generally to *Phosphorus*, *Phosphoric-acid* or *Veratrum.* I have employed them all with success. The *Phosphoric-acid* is to be preferred when there is a gluey matter on the tongue, or cramps in the upper arm or fore-arm or in the wrists or hands, or if the stools are yellowish and the evacuations painless. Give *Phosphorus* when there is a white or brown coat on the tongue and the evacuations attended with griping or colicky pains, or with nausea. Give *Veratrum* when the coat on the tongue is yellow and the diarrhœa painful. In some cases, *Arsenicum*, *Mercurius* or *Secale* may be indicated.

---

* See also Chapter VI, section 1st, for the treatment of its first stage.

However, Phosphor, Phosphoric-acid or Verat., generally cure; and they may often be given at first, without the previous administration of Camphor, in this form of Cholera. When the evacuations are very copious, liquid and frequent, Camphor should not be given so many times before resorting to other medicines. Put two or three globules of the 30th attenuation of *Phosphorus*, or of the 3d attenuation of *Phosphoric-acid*, in a little sugar of milk, and place them on the patient's tongue; or give them in solution, in the manner described in Chapter VI. After two or three doses of Phos-ac. [3], if the indications for Phos.-ac. remain, it will often be useful to employ the 30th. A dose of the appropriate remedy may be given after each evacuation, if it is copious, or every second evacuation, if they are small.

SYMPTOMS OF THE SECOND VARIETY, CHOLERA GASTRICA, GASTRIC CHOLERA.

This form of Cholera is characterized by frequent or almost continual *vomiting*, but is often accompanied by many symptoms of other varieties. The matters at first thrown out consist of the food which the stomach happened to contain, or the liquids which had been swallowed. They are usually thrown up with a sudden jerk, without previous retching. The vomiting is sometimes preceded for a short time by nausea. There is no diarrhœa, or only one or two evacuations at the onset. The urine is scanty.

The gastric variety of Cholera is neither the most frequent nor the most dangerous. When the epidemic prevails, this form may be excited by flatulent vegetables or other indigestible food.

TREATMENT OF GASTRIC CHOLERA.

The principal remedies are *Camphor* and *Veratrum*. *Camphor* will ordinarily be proper at the onset; one drop every five minutes. If relief is not soon obtained, give *Veratrum* ^{12}, at the usual intervals, unless some other remedy is more indicated by the character, conditions or concomitants of the vomiting.* If, by the effect of the Veratrum or Ipecac., the vomiting cease, but the other symptoms remain, and there is great weight at the stomach and pains in the intestines and head, then have recourse to *Nux* ^{30}. But if the disease is not checked, give *Verat.* ^{30}, or other medicines according to the indications. To Cholera excited by anger, and attended with either vomiting to diarrhœa, *Cham.* ^{12} is appropriate.

SYMPTOMS OF THE THIRD VARIETY, CHOLERA SPASMODICA, SPASMODIC CHOLERA.

This form is especially characterized by *cramps* and other *spasms*. The principal symptoms are,

* Examine the repertories to decide between these, or to determine whether some other remedy is preferable.

contractions and cramps in the toes and fingers; afterwards, cramps in the calves, or convulsive movements in the muscles of the fore-arm, and legs; then spasms in the upper arms and thighs, and sometimes fixed spasms in the chest, neck and jaw, resembling those of locked jaw or tetanus. The constriction of the chest is preceded by vomiting. Neither vomiting nor diarrhœa frequently occur in this variety; but it may succeed a neglected diarrhœa, and be ushered in by a single copious vomiting, and attended by occasional retchings.

In some cases, there are first cramps in the calves of the legs; then tonic spasms of the whole of both inferior extremities, soon extending in succession to the abdomen, stomach, chest and throat; the inferior limbs remaining spasmodically extended and extremely stiff and hard, and affected with excruciating pain; a hard swelling at the stomach; spasms of the muscles of the jaw, attended with grating of the teeth; respiration almost arrested; sense of extreme suffocation; apprehension of impending dissolution; deglutition difficult, sometimes impossible. The spasms at length relax, and the patient for a few minutes, is free from pain. Then the spasms and the pain return with their former severity.

TREATMENT OF SPASMODIC CHOLERA.

The principal remedies are *Camphor*, *Cuprum* and *Veratrum*. Give a drop of *Camphor* every five minutes. During the paroxysms, if they are extremely severe, we may give two drops at a dose, or repeat one drop every two or three minutes. The remedy next to be employed for removing the remains of the spasms and preventing their return is ordinarily Cuprum ^{30}. Give it in solution, or dry in doses of two or three globules, and repeat it many times at *intervals* of half an hour, or an hour, if its salutary effect is not manifested. If necessary, then give *Veratrum* (12th then 30th) in repeated doses, or other medicines according to the different indications. Cuprum may be given at the onset of the spasms, provided their character and concomitants indicate its use decidedly more than that of Camphor. Vide Cholera Repertory.

SYMPTOMS OF THE FOURTH VARIETY, CHOLERA SICCA, DRY CHOLERA.

There is *no diarrhœa nor vomiting*. Sometimes the attack is first manifested by a blackish color of certain parts, as the ends of the fingers, whilst the general strength is not seriously impaired. In the severer forms, there is a *sudden prostration* of the vital powers; the urine is suppressed; tongue sometimes blue or blackish; the eyes up-turned and fixed; coldness of the surface of the whole body, which becomes covered with a cold, sticky sweat; the face and limbs have a violet blue color. The voice and pulse fail. This variety requires the most prompt attention.

TREATMENT OF DRY CHOLERA.

The first remedy, as in other varieties of Cholera, is *Camphor*. In this variety, it is especially required, for arousing the nervous system. Repeat it in doses of one or two drops, every five minutes. Then, if necessary, give Veratrum every half hour, or hour, or hour and a half. If the cramps and vomitings have entirely ceased, if the patient is cold, blue and pulseless, i. e. collapsed—*Carbo-v.* ^{30}, two or three globules. In this state of complete asphyxia, some recommend hydrocianic acid, 3d attenuation, every hour or two. We recognise the effect of these medicines by the pulsations becoming sensible, and sometimes by a return of the cramps, vomitings or diarrhœa; symptoms which are then to be treated by *Veratrum* or *Cuprum*, or some other remedy, according to the indication.

SYMPTOMS OF THE FIFTH VARIETY, CHOLERA ACUTA, ACUTE CHOLERA.

In this variety the nervous centres seem to be effected in the first stage. Yet in its course it simulates the form of some other varieties, and like them, unless checked, ends in asphyxia and death.

The patient at first feels as if he were stunned, or has a sensation of weight in the head, or vertigo; oppression of the chest; numbness of the arms and legs. Afterwards there are rumblings in the intestines; heat of the body, pulse rapid and feeble; nausea, retching or vomiting; bilious or watery diarrhœa; suppression of urine; tongue cold; voice altered; face yellowish, with a dark blue circle around the eyes; prostration; spasms, at first, in the feet and hands, afterwards extending to the arms and legs, which become dark-blue and cold; the eyes tarnished and sunk in their orbits. The diarrhœa and cramps cease, and the disease in its later stage runs into the form of dry Cholera, characterized by cold sweats, insensible pulse, and general blueness—i. e. by collapse.

The above descriptions of the dry and acute Cholera, are extracted mainly from the treatise of Dr. F. F. Quin. In both, the strong impression of the poison on the nervous system, seems to produce an unusually great and early change in oxygenation and the constitution of the blood. There is probably no impropriety in applying the term acute to most of those cases which without being dry, are *sudden* in their invasion and *rapid* in their course. Such cases not unfrequently present complications which prevent their being embraced in any other single class, unless we should add a new one to those here enumerated.

TREATMENT OF ACUTE CHOLERA.

Give *Veratrum;* at first the 12th, in persons of vigorous constitution, and after three doses, the 30th, in the quantity and at the intervals before described. In cases of persons of feeble constitution, give one dose of the 12th, and follow it by as many of the 30th as shall be necessary.

If in this or in any other variety of Cholera, there is severe burning in any part of the alimentary-canal, with violent colic, and great weakness or restlessness, give *Arsenicum* ³⁰. If the colic proves obstinate, give an enema of ice-water. Though Veratrum is in general the grand remedy for this somewhat complicated variety, yet it will often be necessary to consult the repertory, and determine the remedy by groups of symptoms.*

SYMPTOMS OF THE SIXTH VARIETY,
CHOLERA GASTRO-ENTERICA,
GASTRO-ENTERIC CHOLERA.

This is a kind of combination of the gastric and diarrhoeic varieties; yet being not unfrequent in its occurrence, it merits a distinct consideration. It is characterized by vomiting and diarrhœa, almost simultaneous in their commencement, and nearly equal in their intensity and duration. These evacuations from the stomach and intestines agree in another respect: viz. in consisting at first of the usual contents of those cavities respectively, (i. e. food being vomited, and fœcal matter dejected,) and in soon be-

* The treatment of the dry and acute varieties, is taken mainly from the treatise of Dr. F. F. Quin of London.

coming thinner, afterwards watery, and ultimately assuming the rice-water appearance. Although this combination of upward and downward discharges is characteristic of this variety, there may be some cramps, and great coldness of the body, and the patient may be, within a few hours after the attack, in the blue and pulseless condition of collapse.

TREATMENT OF GASTRO-ENTERIC CHOLERA.

The principal remedy is *Veratrum*, in the doses and at the intervals before mentioned. If a dose or two of the 12th is given at first, the 30th should be given subsequently.

If the treatment is commenced very early, *Camphor* will be appropriate, and ordinarily sufficient. Dose, one drop every five minutes. When the stools become exceedingly copious and liquid, *Veratrum* is in most cases to be used. If there is complication of other symptoms, the groups may indicate some other remedy.

SYMPTOMS OF THE SEVENTH VARIETY, CHOLERA DYSENTERICA, DYSENTERIC CHOLERA.*

This variety commences with the symptoms of diarrhœic Cholera, and gradually becomes more

* Dr. Quin, from whom the above classification is in part taken, comprises in "Dysenteric Cholera," what is here named Diarrhœic, if he does not restrict it to that.

dysenteric. The diarrhœa from the outset is attended with pain in the abdomen. The stools, copious and watery, presently acquire the rice-water character. After some time they diminish in quantity, and present, in addition to the watery and ricey portions, some mucus, which still later becomes sanguineous, but is still accompanied by ricey and watery portions. If the disease continue some days, the ricey evacuations are replaced by others of bloody mucus or blood. Cramps of the feet may exist early in the second stage, and even precede the attack as a premonitory symptom.

Many cases of dysenteric Cholera occurred in 1849. They were distinguishable from dysentery (many cases of which also occurred in the same epidemic) by the Cholera symptoms which predominated in the earlier stages.

On account of the frequent occurrence of this form as compared with all others of an inflammatory character, and the peculiarity in the treatment required, there is a practical advantage in giving it a distinct consideration and name. It is therefore placed by itself in this edition. It is not usually in any remarkable degree, a febrile disease: the depression of the vital forces by the Cholera proper, seems in many cases to overbalance the general excitement which the associated inflammation of the mucous membrane of the large intestine tends to produce. And this inflammation when uncomplicated, is seldom attended with as much fulness of pulse and pains in various parts, as characterize many other inflammations and fevers. Yet there are cases where this variety is complicated with the succeeding. There may be similar complications in the case of other varieties. I am not insensible to the defects of this and all classifications, of the disease, but deem it practically useful to adopt one that is approximately correct.

TREATMENT OF DYSENTERIC CHOLERA.

The principal remedies for this variety, are *Camphor*, *Veratrum*, *Mercurius-vivus*, and *Sulphur*—in the above order.

There being an inflammation of the mucous membrane of the large intestine, we should make but a sparing and cautious use of Camphor.*

Give three or four doses of *Camphor* ^{3}, at intervals of a quarter or half an hour, or, if this is not at hand, as many quarter-drop doses of the tincture; then *Veratrum* ^{12} or ^{30}, until the evacuations become small and bloody; then *Mercurius* ^{12}, followed after some time by *Mercurius* ^{30}. After amendment of the dysenteric portion of the disease, commences, the cure is to be completed by *Sulphur* ^{30}.

* I think a similar precaution in regard to Camphor, is advisable in treating *children* in cholera *generally*. Nearly all the fatal cases which I have heard of as occurring after an early use of Camphor, have been among children under twelve years of age. I would advise that in the cases of children, Camphor be not employed lower than the third dilution.

Sometimes, when there is inflammatory fever, two or three doses of *Aconite* will be required before the Mercurius, or during a temporary suspension of the use of the latter.

SYMPTOMS OF THE EIGHTH VARIETY, CHOLERA FEBRILIS, FEBRILE CHOLERA.

In some instances, cholera is complicated with fever. This is distinguishable from other febrile diseases, by the watery and ricey evacuations, or the nausea vomitings and spasms; and from other forms of cholera, by the frequency, hardness, and fulness of the pulse. The temperature of the body is generally above the normal standard, that of the hands and feet, sometimes below. Pains in the small of the back, hips, limbs, head, and abdomen. Redness of the eyes, tongue, or fingers.

TREATMENT OF FEBRILE CHOLERA.

In febrile cholera, give but little Camphor. For a short time use Veratrum, or other remedies adapted to the purging vomiting, or cramps, if either is severe. Then Aconitum ^{12} or ^{30} in solution, a dose once in two or three hours, if the pulse is hard, full and rapid, and there is great thirst, and heat of skin. Otherwise use Rhus-radicans ^{30}, for the rheumatic-like pains. This last remedy will be especially indicated if the tip of the tongue is red. Then Bell. ^{30}, Bry. ^{30}, or Canth. ^{30}, according to the symptoms and the organ affected. The accurate selection of the remedy in these cases can be made only by a homœopathic physician.

The foregoing varieties are in some cases well marked, in others not. There is an advantage in attending to them; though the homœopathic physician who prescribes for the symptoms, will not deem it necessary to designate the variety. This will often be impracticable, especially if he is called when the cases are so advanced as to confound varieties which were originally distinct. In one sense, the variety may change with the stage.

CHAPTER VIII.

SYMPTOMS AND TREATMENT OF THE STAGES OF CHOLERA.

A case of either of the foregoing varieties is not usually divisible into distinct, well-defined stages; but we may enumerate four stages; some of them being oftener present or more distinct or durable in one variety, and some in another. They are: 1st. *The incipient Stage*, or *Stage of Invasion:* 2d. *The*

Active Stage, or *Stage of Full Development:* 3d. *The Stage of Collapse:* and 4th. *The Stage of Reaction.*

FIRST STAGE, STAGE OF INVASION.

This is usually longest in the diarrhœic variety; in which it may continue from one hour to several days. The stools, though they may be watery and whitish, are not profuse. In the gastric variety, this stage may present a transient nausea, or a few loose fœcal stools; in the spasmodic variety, diarrhœa, or one or two vomitings; in the acute variety, vertigo; in the gastro-enteric variety, nausea.

When cholera prevails, the above symptoms are generally due to the action of its poison. This is evident from their general prevalence during the epidemic, their amenability to cholera remedies, and the formidable and unequivocal phases which they frequently assume, when nature is unaided.

There are two modes of considering these symptoms—either as constituting a milder form, or an earlier stage. The latter is here preferred. Some of these cases would stop in this stage, others become fully developed, and finally fatal. No power of diagnosis could at first separate them into two classes, founded on their inherent tendencies. Could we distinguish those which would spontaneously prove abortive, we would exclude them, even from the first stage. But that distinction is impracticable. Without any assumption in regard to their nature, the event under treatment, will subsequently decide whether they assume a form more complicated and severe; and as it requires a certain number and severity of symptoms, to constitute the disease in its more formidable and popular sense, we never include in our cholera reports, the cases cured in this stage of invasion.*

The principal *remedies* in the first stage are: *Camphor*, *Phosphorus*, *Phosphoric-acid*, and *Veratrum.*

SECOND STAGE, STAGE OF FULL DEVELOPMENT.

This, in the diarrhœic variety, is characterized by the profuse or frequent rice-water evacuations; in the gastric variety, by the vomiting of similar matter; in the spasmodic variety, by severe cramps or other spasms; in the dry variety, the first two stages may be scarcely perceptible, unless the first is, by the dark color of certain parts, or the coldness of the tongue; in the acute variety, there may be a livid appearance under the eyes, vomiting, or rumblings and liquid stools. In the gastro-enteric variety, there is profuse vomiting and diarrhœa; in the dysenteric varie-

* In an essay published in the appendix to this book, this stage is designated by the convenient term *Choleroid.* This term includes Cholerine, but has the advantage of greater comprehensiveness.

ty, pain and tenderness of the abdomen, and watery, ricey, and bloody-mucous discharges.

The stage of full development has usually one of two terminations; viz., either collapse, or convalescence.

In fully developed cholera, the principal remedies are: *Camphor*, *Veratrum*, *Cuprum*, *Phosphorus*, *Phosphoric-acid*, and *Arsenicum*.

It is the commencement of this stage, that is alluded to in Chapter VI,* as "a decided attack." For the details of its early treatment, the second section of that chapter is to be consulted—also the Repertories.

THIRD STAGE, STAGE OF COLLAPSE.

This stage of collapse may have the same character in every variety of Cholera, and in its principal features it is similar in all varieties. The term collapse is used to designate a certain collection of symptoms, including pulselessness; cold, blue and shrivelled skin; the voice reduced to a whisper; the urine and other secretions suppressed, and the face presenting a certain appearance called Choleric. The term faciës cholerica is used to denote a face cold, livid and shrunk, and often anxious, the eyes sunk in the orbits, and upturned, or fixed, as if in vacant staring. The vox cholerica, which belongs chiefly to

* Page 102.

this stage, is a voice hoarse, feeble, whispering, or almost imperceptible.

The duration of the third stage, varies from two hours to two days. It has one of three terminations; viz., either death, convalescence, or a disease which is inflammatory, congestive, or typhus. When death occurs from Cholera, it is usually at the termination of the third stage, sometimes of the fourth. The return of a perceptible pulse, and of warmth, although attended with a renewal of the vomiting and diarrhœa, are favorable signs; though even after this partial reaction, there may be a relapse into asphyxia.

If the collapse is complete, the principal *remedies* are *Cuprum*, *Arsenicum*, *Carbo-vegetabilis*, and *Secale*. When the collapse is only incipient or partial, *Camphor* and *Veratrum*. These may also be required for a while in complete collapse, if they have not been resorted to in an earlier stage of the same case.

FOURTH STAGE, STAGE OF REACTION AND SECONDARY AFFECTIONS.

The secondary affections which ensue on reaction, are congestive, *inflammatory*, or *febrile*. The fourth stage proper, i. e., reaction attended with these serious diseases, has seldom any existence after a good homœopathic treatment of Cholera proper; though there will, in some cases, be dysuria. The affections to be most apprehended after allopathic treatment, are, inflammation, or congestion of the brain, stomach, intestines, or lungs; or typhoid fever.

So far as there is a partial reproduction of the symptoms of the second stage, which had disappeared during the collapse, a recurrence to the remedies of the second stage will be necessary in the fourth. But for the new symptoms following reaction, use other remedies. For the irritation of the bladder, attended with painful urination, use *Cantharis* [30], every hour or two, whilst the symptoms remain urgent.

In most of these *inflammations*, however, we may give two or three doses of Acon. [24], at intervals of an hour, and then follow it by the remedy adapted to the symptoms, and the organ affected; repeating this last medicine much less frequently. If it is the *brain* that is affected, the remedy will generally be *Belladonna* [30]; if the *lungs*, *Bryonia* [30], in some cases followed by *Rhus* [30]; if the *stomach* or *intestines*, *Nux* [30], and sometimes *Bry.* [30]; if the *bladder*, *Cantharis* [30]. This last is also the remedy where there is inflammation in the lower intestines, attended with burning, tenesmus, and bloody stools. For the typhus or typhoid *fever*, *Bryonia*, and sometimes *Phosphoric-acid*, may be used; but the principal remedy is *Rhus-radicans*.*

* I deem it due to the profession as well as to myself, to state, that the Note on this plant, inserted without my consent or knowledge, in the Appendix to the American edition of Jahr's Sympto-

I will take this occasion to make a remark on a topic, not discussed in either of the notes above referred to. The Rhus-tox. which Hahnemann tried, was an exotic, and hence probably did not possess as much power as a plant of the same species found growing in its native soil in America. Dr. Wallace, a scientific oculist of this city, informs me that this is the case with Stramonium; and that, on the other hand, the Belladonna of Europe is more powerful, in dilating the pupil, than the exotic Belladonna of America. Again, if the shrub Rhus-tox. is a stunted variety of the same species as the vine Rhus-rad., there is an additional reason for doubting whether it has as much activity; furthermore, the provings afford evidence that it has not. So far as the clinical experience of many physicians for some years can show, the Rhus-rad. is as efficacious as Rhus-tox. or more so, in those cases to which the latter is applicable. Like several other physicians, I prefer it. Wherever in the repertory, the generic term *Rhus* is used alone, it may be considered as including both *Rhus-rad.* and *Rhus-tox.*

men-Codex, is grossly incorrect, especially where it attempts to correct my botanical description of this plant in general, and of the particular plant from which I obtained the specimen for trial. This last part of the criticism is not only incorrect, but absurd; inasmuch as the botanical character of those particular leaves could be known only to myself and my respectable medical colleagues who engaged with me in the provings, and to whom the leaves were shown. I here re-affirm the correctness of my description, as given in the Note in the body of the same Symptomen-Codex, pages 671 and 672.

If great debility follows the Cholera, and there are no other symptoms which require special attention, the appropriate remedy is *Cinchona* [12]. The final remedy for the more complete restoration of health, will frequently be Sulph. [30], given in a single dose, and allowed to act a long time without repetition.

When a homœopathic physician is called in any stage, to any case of Cholera which *has been under allopathic treatment*, he is first to antidote the former treatment by *Camphor*. Give it but a short time, if there is any inflammation. He can judge if other antidotes are necessary; as they frequently will be in the course of the treatment; for calomel and crude drugs—and even the undiluted colored tinctures of the homœopathic shops—are so durable in their mischievous action, as to require for their correction, something more durable in its curative action, than Camphor.

CHAPTER IX.

CASES OF CHOLERA IN NEW-YORK,

IN 1849 AND SUBSEQUENT YEARS—WITH A FEW EXAMPLES OF CHOLEROID DISEASE.

PRELIMINARY REMARKS.

The following cases are given as examples of the symptoms and treatment of several forms of the disease. To give them value for statistical use, a report of the entire number of cases would be requisite.

The author regrets, that the engrossing nature of his practice in the epidemic, left him too little time to give as full description even of the cases here published, as would be desirable. The records of most of his other cases are meagre. Some of those here given will be of use to the student and practitioner; they perhaps occupy sufficient space in the book for most practical purposes. The patients were persons of intelligence, and their statements reliable. All the cases except the 5th, 14th, 15th, 18th, and 19th, occurred when the Cholera was extensively prevalent. Some may be disposed to call the rarer cases sporadic. Sporadic means scattered, and is properly and generally applied to cases of disease which are not only scattering, but independent of any epidemic or contagious influence.

When cases occur at long intervals, are few and isolated, some persons doubt whether they are Asiatic Cholera, however characteristic the symptoms—because, say the sceptics, Cholera, when it exists, is an epidemic, i. e., a prevalent disease. But an epidemic must have a beginning and termination, in single cases; and subsequent to the first, and antecedent to the last, are rare cases. By cutting off both ends of the pestilence, pronouncing them sporadic, and thus putting them in another category, some prove to their own satisfaction, from experience, that Cholera when it actually exists, is a prevalent disease.

The next step is to apply this inference in justifying the subsequent exclusion of rare and isolated cases. This is reasoning in a circle.

The term epidemic may be properly employed, either with reference to the general prevalence of the atmospheric, or other invisible cause, or to the general prevalence of the resulting disease. The cause is epidemic (epidemos, upon the people,) earlier than the disease; and, after its introduction, it, or some impression made by it, may exist for years, but in such a state as to produce only a few cases. At different times since 1849, I have seen cases here, which resembled Cholera more strongly than any which had fallen under my observation for many preceding years.

Such considerations are calculated to allay rather than excite, undue apprehension in the public mind, at times when composure is most needful. The idea that a new poison is just now imported, is more dreadful than that of an addition to one previously present. If medical men and municipal officers conceal the scattering cases, and suddenly announce the arrival of the pestilence after it has gained a more formidable strength, the public mind not only receives a severe shock, but at a time when more than at any other, such excitement is dangerous. Besides, such concealment at the earliest and last stages of the epidemic, tends to prevent the adoption of necessary precautions by individuals. I have known of fatal cases which would have been prevented, by information of the existence of Cholera in the city.*

The valuable cases which Drs. Bayard, Quin, and Wright, have reported to the author, are described in the well-selected language of those learned and experienced physicians.

The following cases occurred in the practice of the author, with the exception of those in which the name of some other physician is mentioned in connection with the case. Those which bore some resemblance to Cholera, but wanted a sufficient number or severity of the characteristic symptoms, may be termed Choleroid. It is not considered necessary to give many of these, although in the author's practice, they were about eight times as numerous as the cases reported as Cholera.

Where Camphor was employed in Cholera, it was always, unless otherwise stated, given in drop-doses, in solution in sugared water, prepared according to

* Epidemics seem to depend in some instances, at least in part, upon some cause which increases the predisposition. On this principle, I explain the fact, that the susceptibility to vaccination is greater when small-pox is most prevalent. The latter has at least been the case in this city, during the epidemic small-pox of the winter of 1853–4, as compared with years when the latter disease was far less prevalent. Of the 142 vaccinations performed by me in private practice, from November to March inclusive, more than half were successful, and some in persons who had previously had small-pox, some varioloid, and one in a lady who had had both very decidedly, she now took vaccination in an equally decided degree. Nearly all the subjects had been previously vaccinated once or more.

the method described in this book. In regard to other medicines, where only a single dose of any attenuation was administered, it was about three small globules placed dry on the tongue, by itself, or in sugar or saccharum-lactis. Where a greater number of doses of an attenuated medicine were employed, the method was to dissolve about six small globules in a gill, i. e., half a tumblerful of cold water, and direct the patient to take three teaspoonfuls at a time, as a dose.

The professional reader will understand the character ℞ to signify prescription, or treatment prescribed or commenced by the physician. When a figure is prefixed to the name of the medicine, it signifies the number of doses. The figure at the right of the name of the medicine, and a little above, denotes the attenuation or potency.

CASES OF CHOLEROID DISEASE.

CASE 1.—*Diarrhœic Choleroid.*—On Tuesday, July 10th, 1849, an unmarried gentleman, a merchant, aged about 24, applied to me on account of a simple diarrhœa, and received three powders of Camphor^{3}, to be taken dry, and a powder of Veratrum^{30}, to be taken in solution, in seven doses. He was for the time relieved: but in the latter part of the following day, Wednesday, he used some indigestible food in improper quantity. In the succeeding night, Thursday, 2 A. M., he was suddenly attacked with diarrhœa of a different character. In this last attack the stools were at first thin and brown, afterwards watery and white. Veratrum ^{30}, after each evacuation, relieved him permanently.

Remark.—The suddenness of the attack, the nocturnal invasion, and the watery consistence and milky color of the evacuations, are among the characteristics of Cholera. But others were wanting. The patient was not prostrated, but able to call at my office. This may be considered as a case of Cholerine, i. e., Diarrhœic Choleroid.

CASE 2.—*Spasmodic Choleroid.*—On Sunday morning, August 19th, 1849, a merchant, aged 37 years, had a loose evacuation. Without consulting a physician, he took Veratrum. From his medical associations, I had little doubt that it was some low dilution.

At midnight, he was seized with a chill, or paroxysm of shivering, soon attended with cramps in the jaw and wrists. Being alarmed at these symptoms, he sent a carriage for me as soon as possible. The distance was about a mile. In the mean time, he took tincture of Camphor, which on my arrival at a quarter before two, A. M., had been followed by perspiration.

Prescription, Cuprum ^{30}. He was well the same day, Monday, 20th.

Remarks.—This may be considered as a case of spasmodic choleroid; or in other words, spasmodic cholera arrested in the first stage. It sustained the same relation to developed spasmodic cholera, that cholerine does to developed diarrhœic cholera.

That the cholera poison had some agency in the production of this gentleman's symptoms, I subsequently had additional evidence, in being called on the same day, the 20th, to visit two of his children, attacked with diarrhœic cholera; many liquid and ricey evacuations, some of them copious. One at least had a decidedly cold tongue. The symptoms had commenced on the same day as the premonitory looseness of the father, but not with severity sufficient to excite apprehension in the family, and induce them to seek medical aid.

In such epidemics, several nearly simultaneous attacks in a family are not uncommon.

In the epidemic, there were many instances of slight spasmodic choleroid. Thus the cholera poison manifested its influence by exciting frequently repeated cramps in individuals, for several weeks before they were attacked with cholera. Such cases show an early impression on the nervous system. That this impression may be instrumental in changing the blood, and be one of the earliest links in the chain, I long since recognized in an article which was published in the Transactions of the Medical Society of the State of New York, and from which I have extracted most of the first two chapters of this book. It was not thought necessary to extract these more hypothetical parts on pathogeny, and they are referred to now to show, that the nervous theory of cholera is neither new nor incompatible with that given in this book.

In some instances, the change of color of the blood in certain parts, was the most marked of the early symptoms, and almost the only one One of the cases of this kind of *dry choleroid*, which came under my observation, is described in the appendix. It occurred in a young gentleman, at that time laboriously engaged in practising in the epidemic. He was exposed to many of the most malignant cases, and in the most unhealthy localities. The bluish-black color of his fingers, which he describes, I saw several times.

CASE 3.—*Diarrhœic Choleroid.*—On Tuesday, Sept. 25th, 1849, at 8½ A. M., Capt. C. called on me to visit his wife immediately. Aged about 27; had slight diarrhœa last evening. This morning was suddenly attacked with nausea, violent diarrhœa and severe pains in the abdomen. There were three stools, brown and "watery"—two of them large.

℞—3 Veratrum ^{30}, one every hour; afterwards,

only once in three hours, unless there should be evacuations.

Called in the evening, and found that she had immediately recovered under the Veratrum ^{30}.

CASE 4.—M., a girl aged 10. Attacked with violent diarrhœa and colic, in the night, between two and three, A. M., Friday, Sept. 28th, 1849. I was sent for at seven, and arrived at seven and a half, A. M. Five stools, the first three about a pint each, watery, with pea-sized pieces of something yellowish.

℞—1 Arsenicum ^{30}, dry, then Veratrum ^{30}, in solution; each hour till relieved; then once in two hours. Recovery on the same day under the Veratrum ^{30}.

CASE 5.—*Gastro-enteric Choleroid.*—On Thursday, July 21st, 1853, at nine, A. M., B. F. Joslin, Jr., M.D., was called to visit a boy, æt. seven years, who had vomiting and diarrhœa. Had been attacked about four, A. M. The discharges frequent, extremely so at first; most of them yellowish and watery, the last colorless, having the appearance of clear water. Rice-water vomiting; pulse 138; tongue whitish and cool; lips cold. Three hours afterwards, at twelve o'clock, I visited the patient in consultation. There was no vomiting nor diarrhœa. Some degree of reaction had taken place. Arsenicum ^{30} continued. At half past four, P. M.,

Dr. Joslin, Jr., made his third visit. Pulse, 120 and full; lips warm; tongue warm.

℞. Aconitum ^{30}, alternately with Arsenicum ^{30}. On the next day, the boy was found cured. Treatment discontinued.

Remark.—This case approximated very nearly to developed Cholera, but was not reported.

CASE 6.—*Dry Choleroid.*—In the epidemic of 1849, Dr. B., aged 42, was suddenly awakened in the night with a sensation of great coldness. At first he supposed that the wind was blowing upon him. His wife remarked, "you are covered with a profuse, cold sweat." The Doctor then, on examination, perceived that the sweat was general, cold and clammy. Great weakness, with a degree of restlessness. Mrs. B., asked the Doctor what medicine he would take. He replied the third of Camphor. His wife fearing this was not sufficiently powerful, endeavored to persuade him to take the tincture in drop doses. But the Doctor, supposing he had Cholera-sicca, and having reasons to believe in the power of attenuated Camphor, when properly indicated, determined to try it on his own person, and accordingly took a few pellets of the third dilution, i. e. Camph. ^{3}, dry, on the tongue, and after waiting fifteen minutes, repeated the dose. A short time after this, he was conscious of an increased warmth, a drying up of the sweat, which rapidly took place, and a calmness of feeling, which predisposed to sleep. He awoke in the morning with his usual amount of health.

Remark.—This case is placed in the Choleroid class, not because there is any doubt respecting its cause or tendency, but because the disease was arrested in the first stage. Yet the most marked symptom which was present, belongs oftener to the third stage of Cholera of other varieties. The first stage of Cholera-sicca, may be as dangerous as the second or third of some other varieties.

CASES OF DIARRHŒIC CHOLERA.

CASE 7.—On Monday, June 4th, 1849.—Mr. S., a mechanic, aged forty, residing in the upper part of the city, dined later than usual, on stewed kidneys, of which he made his meal. The night following, he was disturbed several times in his sleep by a diarrhœa, with colic before evacuation. The next day, June 5th, it increased; and on the morning following, June 6th, feeling more unwell, he sent for Edward Bayard, M. D. He found the patient vomiting and purging; profuse watery discharges without smell or color; cold sweat over the body, more particularly on the forehead; skin shriveled and blue; tongue and breath cold; pulse scarcely perceptible at the wrist; throwing his arms about with excessive restlessness; complaining of cramps in the region of the stomach and in the calves of his legs; voice sepulchral. Dr. Bayard gave him a drop of the tincture of Camphor in a tablespoonful of water, every fifteen minutes for three times, which produced no visible effect. He then dissolved a few pellets of the thirtieth dynamization of Veratrum in a tumbler one third full of water, and gave a tablespoonful of the mixture, and in thirty minutes repeated the remedy. The pulse rose, and likewise the temperature of the body. On the third dose, the vomiting became frothy, indicative of the action of the medicine. The remedy was then discontinued. In a short time, reaction fully set in, and in a few days, the patient was entirely restored to health.

CASE 8.—On Monday, June 25th, 1849.—A married gentleman, a merchant, aged about 30, was attacked in the night, about two, A. M., with violent watery diarrhœa. When first visited in haste, early in the morning, he had had several evacuations, attended with cold perspiration on the face. Decidedly dark and unnatural color of the face. Great prostration, was unable to step without assistance. Cramps in the abdomen. The watery evacuations still continued. He was treated by Camph. $\frac{1}{10}$, in drop doses, in sugared water, and Camph. ^{3} in solution. The diarrhœa immediately stopped under the Camphor; but Veratrum ^{30}, in solution, was given in the evening and next day. During his convalescence on this second day, he also took one Belladonna ^{30}, and one Nux-vom. ^{1000}, and finally, on the third day, one Nux-vom. ^{30} all dry.

CASE 9.—Friday, June 29th, 1849.—A married lady, aged about 35, had a sudden attack of diarrhœa three days since. She took Camphor tincture, in one drop doses, and being relieved, did not think it necessary to send for a physician. Yesterday walked much. This morning at six o'clock, was attacked with diarrhœa and colic.

I saw her at eleven, A. M. The diarrhœa continued up to that time. In the five hours, she has had twelve stools, I saw the last, which consisted of about three gills of rice-water liquid, with abundant white ricey flocks. Coat on the tongue whitish with a scarcely perceptible tinge of yellow. Urine suppressed.

℞. Phosphorus ^{30}, one dose dry, the others in solution.

Saw her again about four, P. M. She had in one hour considerable cramp in the abdomen, between the umbilicus and right groin; is now free from it. Has taken the Phos. ^{30} every second hour, i. e. three times in all. No stool since commencing it. Is much better. Has had one moderate discharge of urine. Is to take a few more doses of Phos. ^{30}, solut. at intervals of two hours.

Was seen on the next day, but required no repetition of the medicine.

Sunday, the third day. Took one China ^{30}, for the remaining debility.

Tuesday, the fifth day. Convalescent. Took one Sulphur ^{30}.

CASE 10.—Tuesday, July 3d, 1849.—Mrs. C., aged about 32, had had more than forty stools in thirty-six hours. Had taken of her own accord, six one-drop doses of Camphor, and twelve more this evening at intervals of five minutes. At eleven and a quarter, P. M., I was called in great haste, and at eleven and a half found her. Nausea, with much effort avoided vomiting. The diarrhœa continued; the stools liquid. Pain and tenderness of the abdomen, in which were rumblings of gas and sound of running liquid. She had suffered much pain there on both days. The noises in the abdomen had commenced at the midnight preceding the attack, and after unusual fatigue on the preceding day. Feet cold; hands cool. Transient chilliness alternating with heat. She has felt unusually cold this season.

Prescription.—One Verat.^{12} dry, then Verat.^{30} in solution, a dose after each evacuation.

The nausea was for a few minutes increased after the Veratrum ^{12}. Normal warmth returned to the feet soon after its administration.

Wednesday, 11¾ A. M., the third day of the disease, and the second of my treatment.

After one dose of Verat. ^{12}, there has been no stool till this morning, when there were two, but of a very different character from the former, i. e. not liquid, but merely soft. Tenderness of abdomen much relieved—now but slight. Feet cold. The patient feels greatly prostrated—requires the recumbent posture.

Ordered beef broth, and solution of Veratrum ^{30}, *pro re nata*, as *before.*

On the following day, the patient was convalescent. Verat. ^{30} was once more prescribed, and the recovery was completed under its action.

CASE 11.—Thursday, July 5th, 1849.—An unmarried lady, aged about 25, had between midnight and noon, when I saw her, twelve, or more, liquid stools, varying in quantity from a pint to a quart each; the first brownish. Those in the morning had the rice-water character. She described them as containing numerous small white pieces, like the curds of milk that sometimes pass an infant's bowels. Her extremities were cold in the night; and there were cramps in the calves of the legs. She took ten doses of Camphor, one drop each.

Her pulse is now weak and slow.

Prescription.—Verat. ^{30} in solution, once in two hours.

Six, P. M. Much better. No evacuations since commencing the Veratrum.

Friday, the second day. The patient is weak. Prescription: China ^{24}, twice a day, three doses.

On the fourth and fifth day of the disease, she again took Veratrum ^{30} in solution. The recovery was completed without any farther prescription.

Remarks. The cure seems to have been principally effected by Camph. $\frac{1}{10}$ and Veratrum ^{30}. The effect of China is not stated in the record. Debility, when caused by profuse evacuations, as it seemed to be in part in this case, is one of the indications for its use.

CASE 12.—A married lady, aged 34, was attacked on Thursday, Aug. 23d, 1849, in the morning, but not visited till next day at half past five, P. M., when she had had thirty alvine evacuations. The aggregate measure of the stools was about three gallons. In consistence and color many, if not most of them, resembled milky water or rice-water. The patient had but little pain, and no apprehension of danger, but expressed merely her astonishment, that the contents of the bowels should pass from her "like a flood." The pulse was extremely feeble, and the tongue cold.

The Cholera prevailed much in the immediate neighborhood, and many deaths had just occurred there.

Now commenced Veratrum ^{30} in solution, to be repeated every hour. My son, B. F. J., Jr., saw her in the evening, and continued the Verat. ^{30}.

Saturday, the third day. At half past ten o'clock, last night, the patient had a rice water and ricey stool, measuring two quarts. The next evacuation occurred at one, A. M., and showed, by the quantity and color, a decided improvement, the stool measured but one pint, and was yellowish. Since that there has been none. The tongue is warm. Prescribed Veratrum ^{30}, in solution, once in two hours.

On Sunday, the fourth day, the patient was found convalescent, but the Verat. ^{30} was given again that day. She recovered without the use of any other medicine, in any stage of the treatment.

Remarks.—The total amount of the evacuations was nearly four gallons. I saw no fatal case, in which there was good evidence of as great a quantity of liquid being discharged, as in this. The more important changes in the blood seem to be more dependent upon the impression made by the poison on the nervous system, than upon the loss of its more liquid portions consequent upon evacuations; though in many constitutions, a copious discharge, as compared with a moderate one, will, *cæteris paribus*, result from a stronger impression. But in the severest asphyxial cases, the impression is too strong to admit of much if any evacuation.

CASE 13.—On Sunday, Sept. 16th, 1849, the owner and superintendent of a manufacturing establishment, aged 34, had a loose evacuation in the morning. In the course of the day was somewhat thirsty. I saw him and prescribed Veratrum ^{30}. About ten o'clock in the evening, he had a sudden and loose movement of the bowels, preceded by a sense of oppression at the stomach. Afterwards in the night there were five brown and liquid stools, each measuring about a pint and a half. The desire to evacuate was urgent and irresistible; and the evacuations attended with rumblings and nausea. Pain and tenderness in the stomach, but none in the abdomen. No sleep in the night.

Monday, the second day, at noon.

Urine has been almost or quite suppressed. The patient passed about a gill and a half, after eight and a half hours. Prostrated—keeps his bed. The nausea, tenderness of the stomach, and diarrhœa continue. The last two stools were examined and found to be quite watery. The evacuations excited by any movement of the body.

Treatment.—Phosphoric-acid ^{30} given in solution, every third hour.

Tuesday, the third day.

Convalescent. No stool after commencing the Phosphoric-acid ^{30}. Tongue warm; red at the tip. Medicine was then discontinued.

Wednesday, the fourth day.

Relapse.—The patient had gone out prematurely, had eaten a peach, a potato, and soup containing tomatos and other vegetables. Had had some nausea on this and the day previous, but had not considered it worth mentioning. At ten o'clock this evening, a profuse diarrhœa commenced suddenly; had four evacuations, above two quarts in all, in an hour and a quarter. Sent immediately for medical aid. I I saw him at eleven, P. M., and examined the stools; they were liquid and brown. Nausea. Anterior part of nose cold. Tongue not cold; neither were the feet. Pulse slow, 54. *Prescribed* Veratrum ^{30}, one dose dry; this was repeated in solution, after the next evacuation, which occurred in about half an hour after the preceding. About the same time had a sensation of general chilliness.

Quarter before twelve, P. M.

Tongue perfectly cold at the anterior part; nose still cold; restlessness. Pain at upper part of stomach, since this last attack. Prescribed one dose of Arsenicum ^{30}, at this time, quarter before twelve o'clock.

Quarter past twelve o'clock, at night.

No evacuation since the second dose of Verat. ^{30}. Tongue became warm, half an hour after the first dose of Arsenicum ^{30}. The patient was then left, with directions to take Veratrum ^{30} and Arsenicum ^{30}, alternately after each evacuation, or in any case at intervals of one and a half hours, if awake. Should there be extensive coldness of the body, Carbo.-veg. ^{30}, was to be administered.

Thursday, the fifth day.

Eleven, A. M. One copious stool in the night, and one this morning: they were like the preceding ones in color and quantity, but still thinner—quite watery. Has taken the Verat. ^{30} and Arsen. ^{30}, alternately. Tongue warm; slight tenderness of the stomach and abdomen; movement in the abdomen, sounding like the trickling of a liquid; pains in the temples, sharp but not shooting. Prescribed Veratrum ^{30} in solution.—The patient recovered under this medicine.

Remark.—Relapses during convalescence are to

be carefully guarded against, by avoiding errors of diet and undue exertion.

CASE 14.—In 1854, on Sunday, May 7th, at three, P. M., Clark Wright, M. D., was called to visit a merchant of this city, who was suffering under Cholera, having been attacked in the previous night, at two, A. M. The family and patient gave the following description of the case.

He was suddenly attacked with diarrhœa; the stools liquid and profuse. The evacuations continued at intervals, up to the time of the first visit. The patient expressed his astonishment at the quantity, wondering "where so much could come from."

At three, P. M., Dr. W. found the pulse very feeble; extremities cold; cramps in the calves and thighs; skin of the hands inelastic, and that of the fingers corrugated; an unnatural, hoarse, and hollow voice; bluish tinge of the face, and dark color under the eyes.

Soon after this, there was another evacuation. The stool on examination, was found to be serous with whitish flocks. Urine extremely scanty. There had been no treatment.

There was now prepared a solution of Camphor, made by dropping six drops of the tincture on a lump of sugar, and dissolving this in two-thirds of a tumblerful of water. Dose, a table-spoonful, once in from five to ten minutes, for an hour. Then, when there began to be more warmth in the extremities, and some improvement in the pulse, the Camphor was discontinued, and a dose of Veratrum [6] given.

About an hour afterwards, there was an evacuation, like dirty rice-water, followed by extreme prostration and thirst; also, nausea and sensation of sinking at the stomach; and profuse and cool perspiration. Drowsiness, with eyes half closed and eye-balls upturned.

Ice was then given, *ad libitum*, and Camphor resumed in the same doses as before, i. e. half a drop each, and given every five minutes, for half an hour, when the perspiration became warm. It soon afterwards dried up, leaving the skin warm. Camphor then stopped. Veratrum [6], and Phos.-acid [12], then given alternately, every half hour. Two doses of each were taken.

The patient then fell into a sweet sleep, slept for half an hour, and awoke refreshed. Had another but smaller passage, slightly tinged with yellow, afterwards another of a deeper yellow.

After waiting two hours, there being no stool, and all other symptoms improving, Dr. Wright made the following prescription for the night: Verat. [6] and Phosphorus [6] alternately, one after every stool.

Monday, second day, in the morning. Had had only two stools and taken two doses. The last, which had been saved, had a fœcal odor.

In the course of the day, had three stools of more consistence, and a more natural color.

On Tuesday, the third day, the medicine was discontinued, and the patient took gruel with more appetite.

On Wednesday, the fourth day, he walked out.

Remarks.—There was occasionally a case of Cholera in the city, about this time, but no reports of them were published. In respect to want of prevalence this case was sporadic; but it was evidently of the same nature as the Asiatic or epidemic Cholera. There was no known occasional cause, nor any thing in the habits of the patient to which the disease could be attributed. I am of opinion, that the poison, in a dilute form, is among us.

CASE 15.—In 1854, on Sunday, May 21st, at four o'clock in the morning, a lady was suddenly attacked with diarrhœa, after having eaten, on the previous day, Rhubarb pie at dinner. Had several very large, watery and lightish brown stools, "as though" she "had taken a large dose of Calomel." Frequent but smaller stools during the day. She again eat a piece of Rhubarb pie.

On the next morning, Monday, the diarrhœa resumed its original violence at the hour corresponding to that of the primary attack, four, A. M. The lady had, at that hour, a return of the copious and watery evacuations. Through the day, Monday the second day, had smaller ones of the same watery character, more frequent after eating. Face pale. Eat freely of rice-pudding. About ten o'clock in the evening, at the suggestion of a physician who was visiting one of the family, she took Bi-carbonate of Soda, in table-spoonful doses of a solution made by dissolving a tea-spoonful of this salt in two thirds of a tumblerful of water; which was to be given two or three times, and followed by one-drop doses of tincture of Camphor after each evacuation. She took these during the night; five doses of the former and fifteen of the latter. After three of the Soda and several of the Camphor, becoming worse, and attributing this to the want of sufficient Soda, she took two more doses, but without improvement; then continued the Camphor°, as before. The Camphor on sugar producing nausea, she afterwards took it in water, recollecting that I had thus prepared it for her father. After this change in the preparation, she experienced no nausea from the Camphor. The diarrhœa, as on previous nights, worse at and after four o'clock; stools individually less copious than in the preceding night, but more numerous and more watery and colorless. These last features excited no alarm, as she thought they might arise from some salutary action of the Camphor. The diarrhœa continued during the night and morning, at intervals on an average of less than half an hour, up to the time of my first visit and prescription of *potentized* Camphor. Stools whitish and watery, some colorless, some like milk mixed with an equal quantity of a solution of coffee, others like water containing yellowish white curd-like sediment. Awake nearly the whole night, when sleep commenced being almost immediately awoke by the diarrhœa or the premonitory pain in the abdomen. In addition to the ordinary pains, there were at times abdominal cramps. About six times in the night, had intolerable cramps in the calves of the legs, a symptom which she had never before experienced in any degree, in any part of the legs, except during an attack of Cholera in the epidemic of 1832.

On Tuesday morning, the third day, at nine o'clock, I, being her physician, was requested to visit her immediately, and called in a quarter of an hour. The patient and her servants were forcibly struck with the great change in her complexion, the very dark color of her face and hands. I found her face and hands of an unnaturally dark color, and the skin of the hands much wrinkled, and so inelastic as to retain for a considerable time any folds into which it was drawn or pinched up with the fingers. Lips decidedly bluish; pulse small, feeble and eighty-four. Sensation of general coldness, as if the body were exposed to a cool breeze; this coldness more this morning than previously. The watery diarrhœa continued; the same frequency of evacuations. Sensation of dryness of the mouth and throat; desires drink often, but in small quantities. I immediately administered a few dry pellets of Camphor ^{30}, and prepared three other similar doses to be given once in half an hour, also a solution of Arsenicum ^{30}, to be commenced at noon, one hour after the last dose of Camphor, and repeated hourly. After two doses of the 30th of Camphor she felt decidedly better, I perceived that the skin of the face and hands had greatly improved in color, and that of the latter had lost much of of its corrugation. After commencing this medicine, in this attenuated form, the patient was exempt from diarrhœa for about two and a half hours—a respite unprecedented during this illness. No stool until about noon, a few minutes after taking the first dose of the 30th of Arsenicum. The stools in the afternoon and evening were only about half a gill each, being scarcely one-fourth as great as previously, though they were passed at about the same intervals, and were still liquid, but of a browner and more normal color. Pulse 74, still rather feeble. Some pains in the abdomen each time after taking beef broth, the diet and drink used through the day.

I saw her a quarter before nine in the evening, when she felt much better than in the morning, but still feeble, and complained of aching and sensation of fulness in the anterior part of the head. I advised a little ice-water, the drinking of which was immediately followed by a warm but partial perspiration, confined to the forehead, face, chest, hands and arms. This sweat being warm, and being the first instance, since the attack, of moisture appearing on the skin, was, though partial, a somewhat favorable sign. But the evidences of congestion of the brain still remaining, and several symptoms including some of the particular localities of the headache and perspiration, also indicating Camphor, and the small, brownish, watery stools still recurring at the same short intervals, I determined to resume its use in the form of the same dynamization which had proved so effectual in arresting the evacuations in the forenoon; and accordingly, a few minutes after nine o'clock, prescribed four doses of the 30th potency, to be taken, in the form of dry pellets, at intervals of a quarter of an hour—i. e., 4 Camph. ^{30}, $\frac{1}{4}$ h.

After resuming this medicine, she had only two stools, one a quarter before, the other a quarter after ten o'clock, that evening, the former a gill, the latter a table-spoonful, the color and consistence unchanged. The aching and fulness of the head was removed; the patient became comfortable, and soon fell into a sound sleep, which continued through the whole night. Had no return of the evacuations. Next morning she awoke perfectly comfortable, and, at the time of my visit at ten o'clock, was sitting in a chair, and presenting her usual appearance of blooming health. After the half ounce evacuation, which in about a quarter of an hour had followed the last dose of potentized Camphor, given on the previous evening, the convalescent patient had no stool whatever for twenty-four hours, then a small one of natural color and fair consistence.

GASTRIC CHOLERA.

CASE 16.—A nephew of Madame Hahnemann, and son of Mr. D'H., 16 months old, still at the breast, awoke out of sleep at 12 o'clock, on the night of the 15th of June, 1849, with vomiting, forcibly ejecting the contents of the stomach "with a jerk." This vomiting was repeated every few minutes, for about an hour and a half, becoming more watery, until it appeared like pure water. Edward Bayard, M.D. saw the patient at one o'clock that night. Eyes sunken, with dark, bluish circles around them; features pinched. Relaxation and heaviness over the whole body; extreme languor, with total apathy except at the time of vomiting. Marbly cold sweat on the face and upper parts of the body, with dryness of the feet and legs. The mother, after consulting Dr. Joslin's book, had administered five one-drop doses of Camphor, at intervals of five minutes.

Dr. Bayard believing that the child was oppressed by the power of the drug, determined to wait for the reaction for thirty minutes. About the expiration of that time, the mother remarked that the child was dying; and it was evident that the symptoms were becoming more intense. The Doctor believing that Camphor was still indicated, determined to give the third dilution, of which he had a few pellets in his box. Three dry pellets of this dilution were placed upon the child's tongue. He vomited once after taking it; the vomiting then ceased. In thirty minutes the dose was repeated. The sweat dried up, the apathy and languor passed away; and in an hour after taking the first dose, the child rose up and played. So convinced was the mother, that her child had been plucked as it were from the jaws of death, by the small dose, that she fell upon her knees and thanked God for the gift of Homœopathia.

CASE 17.—An unmarried gentleman, a merchant, aged 25, was attacked on Monday morning, July 9th, 1849. The first symptom was vomiting with coldness of the feet, legs and face. Vomiting, without nausea; a whitish, grey liquid, like prepared starch, containing white flocks, spirted out violently. After two vomitings, he had one loose stool, then two more vomitings. According to previous instructions, he immediately resorted to Camphor, in drop doses, and continued it every five minutes, until he received Veratrum ^{30}, that is until the messenger could bring it from my office, a mile and a half distant. I called on him at eleven, A. M., and found his tongue, feet, legs and forehead cold. Severe pain in the abdomen. Urine suppressed. After the Veratrum ^{30}, which he had taken, I gave, in the following order: 2 Verat. ^{12}, 1 Nux-vom. ^{30}, 2 Arsenicum ^{30}, and 1 Verat. ^{12}. Then, the more urgent symptoms being relieved, I prescribed Verat. ^{30}, in solution, at one-hour intervals, as long as necessary.

On the day after that of the attack, he was so far restored, that the Veratrum ^{30}, was ordered only three times a day, to be taken for two days if necessary. No other visit or prescription was needed; but I ascertained on the fifth day, that the recovery had been complete under the Veratrum ^{30}, probably in less than three days from the time of attack.

SPASMODIC CHOLERA.

CASE 18.—After having for a week or two a watery diarrhœa, without treatment or medical advice, a married lady was attacked with Cholera of the Spasmodic variety, about half-past nine o'clock in the evening of Monday, January 29th, 1849. I saw her in an hour from the time when the disease assumed this form.

After a single vomiting of some sour material, the patient was attacked with spasms, first as cramps in the calves of the legs; then severe tonic spasms of the whole of both inferior extremities; these tonic spasms, soon extending upwards, successively to the abdomen, stomach, chest and throat. The paroxysms recur simultaneously in the muscles of all those regions, from the legs to the throat, inclusive. The inferior limbs are spasmodically extended and extremely stiff and hard, and affected with excruciating pain.

Among the other results of spasms, there are present; a hard swelling at the stomach, respiration almost arrested, sense of extreme suffocation, and deglutition difficult, sometimes impossible. The spasms relax, and after a few minutes return with the same severity. Lastly, spasms of the muscles of the jaw, attended with grating of the teeth.

℞. Tincture of Camphor, one or two drops, given in sugared water, every five minutes, until there was a diminution of the spasms; then 2 Cuprum-metallicum ^{30}, at intervals of half an hour. Afterwards, there being retching, and vomiting of a very small quantity of froth, there was given, 1 Verat. ^{12}, and 3 Verat. ^{30}, all at intervals of one and a half hours.

The 3 Verat. ^{30}, were given in solution, and by the friends, during the night, the patient being so much improved, as no longer to require the constant attendance of a physician.

Next morning, Tuesday, the second day, the patient feels comfortable, with the exception of a sensation of soreness. This was undoubtedly an effect of the spasms. A few more doses of Verat. ^{30}, were given on that day, at intervals of two hours. The patient having recovered, no other medicine was given.

Remarks.—The Cholera had been reported the preceding month, but was not prevalent until the latter part of the ensuing spring.—This was the first case in 1849. The poison in the atmosphere was probably very dilute in this cold season, yet was sufficient with some peculiar constitution of the patient and after a week or two of diarrhœa, to develope the disease. This, and the two following, all spasmodic, are the only winter cases of Cholera, which have come under my observation. From such an experience I conjecture, that the cold season is less unfavorable to the development of the spasmodic than of other forms of Cholera.

CASE 19.—A young unmarried man, recently engaged in painting, was attacked with *Spasmodic Cholera*, on Tuesday, Feb. 27th, 1849, about five o'clock in the evening. Feeling, at first, spasms in the shoulder, he took an allopathic dose of tartar emetic; in an hour or two he vomited; then had a few loose stools; then vertigo, and considerable deafness; then tonic spasms, excited and increased by movement of the parts. The spasms commenced in the calves, and extended to the whole inferior extremities, the abdomen, and the stomach. Painful tonic spasms rendered the lower limbs inflexible. The vertigo and deafness continued with the spasms. The patient was deaf more especially to the sound of his own voice, the hearing of which seemed to him prevented by the rumbling of his voice in his head. Great thirst. Vomiting once more of a watery liquid with mucus, part of the ejected liquid being of a milky white color. The fluid spirted from the mouth to the distance of about two yards, as estimated in a horizontal direction. The spasms continued, with marbly coldness of the feet, chin, nose, and tongue; face bluish-pale.

Treatment and effects.—Tincture of Camphor in five doses, too large, and at intervals too long, had been given by the family, in about eighty minutes that elapsed before my arrival. These were without apparent effect. I gave a single drop dissolved in sugared water, once in five minutes. The spasms were in some degree mitigated in two hours after the first administration of Camphor, or forty minutes after commencing the use of it in small doses—of which eight were given. Then Cuprum ^{30} was given, in doses of three globules each, in a dry state. The first dose of Cuprum produced a very decided mitigation of the spasms, restored warmth to the chin, and prevented the recurrence of the vomiting. Two more doses of this medicine at intervals of an hour, removed the spasms entirely. Another dose of it was given an hour afterwards to prevent their return. The spasms never returned. No real diarrhœa occurred till next morning, when there were two watery stools, for which was given Verat. ^{30}, in solution. The patient, when visited on that morning, (Wednesday, the 2d day,) was already sitting up, and feeling comfortable. The last dose of Veratrum was taken on the following morning, Thursday, the 3d day, when he was well.

Cause.—I believe this case of spasmodic cholera to have required for its development the presence, in the atmosphere of our city, of some portion of that poison which in a warmer season would have rendered the disease in some form epidemic. The case in the previous month had convinced me that this cause was among us. Nearly all of the symptoms of the present case are those of epidemic cholera, and some of them peculiarly characteristic. The deafness, however, is not usual. The patient for about a week had been engaged in painting window-blinds, and in that occupation had been exposed to the influence of green paint, the basis of which was copper. He may have absorbed a sufficient quantity of this to aid the inception, and have taken enough of tartar emetic to produce an exacerbation of a disease, which from the action of the essential cause alone, i. e., the atmospheric poison, would not have occurred in any degree which would have justified us in considering and reporting it as a case of Asiatic Cholera. We know that even when the disease is epidemic, the attack of an individual usually requires both a predisposing and an occasional cause, in addition to that essential cause which imparts to the symptoms their peculiar character.

CASE 20.—This was somewhat more complicated than the two preceding, yet as the spasms in their severity, extent, and persistence, were prominent symptoms, it may properly enough be considered as belonging to this variety. As I deemed it my duty, though not required by law at that season, to keep the authorities apprised of the occurrence of any such case, although it might be so far as I knew sporadic, I reported it to the Mayor. As most of my records of this case are mislaid, I extract the following from a copy of the letter which relates to it.

"NEW-YORK, Feb. 21st, 1850.

SIR,—I hereby report one case of Cholera. The

patient is ——, a collector, aged 64 years. As this case occurs so early in the year, that you might doubt its genuineness, I think it proper to mention some of its characteristics. Diarrhœa; vomitings; severe cramps in the fingers, arms, toes, legs, thighs, and chest; urine scanty, now suppressed; coldness and blueness of the skin; anterior part of the tongue cold as marble. Attack at eight o'clock last evening, No medical treatment for more than twelve hours. I was applied to at eight this morning, sent medicine, and saw him at nine. The evacuation which I saw, was entirely like rice-water, with a sediment of white particles, like boiled rice."

The patient was in such pain and jeopardy, collapse being imminent, if not already commenced, that he was visited five times on this, second day. The treatment was Cuprum ^{30}, Camphor ^{3}, and Veratrum ^{30}, in solution. They were given in the above order, but not alternately. The patient being improved, was left with directions to continue the same solution, Veratrum ^{30}. The next morning, Friday the third day of the disease, and the second of the treatment, the patient was found convalescent, and directed to take Veratrum ^{30}, only morning and evening. On the following day, Saturday, the fourth of the disease, and the third of the treatment, he was so far recovered, as to take only one dose of Veratrum ^{30}. The treatment was then discontinued, and the result reported at the earliest opportunity—Monday morning.

Note.—One object in being thus careful to report the existence of every case, and the result, was to contribute my share towards giving the authorities all the information requisite for their guidance, in reference to their hygienic functions; another was to give them the means of verifying the reports, and thus to render the latter more official and reliable in statistics. In the present case, however, the season of the year rendered the former object less important; and the latter object has not yet been subserved by it, as the statistics given in this book include no cases occurring since 1849.

DRY CHOLERA.

CASE 21.—On the night of Tuesday, June 26th, 1849, about 11 o'clock, Capt. W., an unmarried man, aged about 28, was attacked. For about three or four weeks he had been living very freely, having just returned from sea. For some days he had been eating as well as drinking to excess. Was visited by James M. Quin, M. D., at midnight. The Doctor found that the patient had been seized with *vomiturition without vomiting*, and *urgent disposition to stool, without stool.* In this condition he was brought by his attendants, from an out-building to bed, at which time he was seen by the Doctor. His pulse was full, bounding, and 110. The head excessively hot, with great mental distress and anxiety. The rest of the body, especially the extremities, were characteristically cold and clammy, tongue and breath cold. The calves of the legs were very much cramped, and the belly was filled with horrible tormina; the patient writhed into every possible position, from excess of agony.

The treatment, which lasted from that time until four o'clock in the morning, at which time the patient was convalescent, consisted of the tincture Camphor, and Veratrum of the sixth attenuation, internally and externally, of bottles of hot water applied extensively to the body, particularly to the calves of the legs and the inside of the thighs. Another point to which the bottles of hot water were applied, was immediately over the kidneys. As a verification of the correctness of this application, the first permanent relief which the patient experienced was signalized by a copious emission of pale watery urine. At first the treatment consisted of Camphor tincture alone, a drop every three minutes for about the first half hour, and for the next, every five minutes. This remedy, besides its specific character, was particularly adapted to the patient's then existing condition of brain. The cramps in the calves of the legs, however, continuing with unabated violence, indicated strongly the use of Veratrum; and under the use of this remedy, the cramps in the calves of the legs subsided in less than thirty minutes, and a profuse warm perspiration broke out over the whole body. From this moment the patient got rapidly better, and the medicines were continued, but at considerably lengthened intervals. Dr. Quin left him at four o'clock, having been incessantly with him for four hours. Up to this time, *no evacuation by the bowels had taken place.* The patient slept from this time till about noon, when he had a natural, soft, but consistent stool.

ACUTE CHOLERA.

CASE 22.—Attack, Monday, May 28th, 1849.—The patient, a married woman, aged 45, was not seen until she had been suffering for nearly four hours from an attack of severe Cholera, unpreceded by any premonitory diarrhœa. The case then presented the appearance of a combination of the spasmodic and gastro-enteric varieties. It appears from the description of Cholera-acuta, as given by Dr. F. F. Quin, and to a considerable extent copied in this book, that this variety, in its second stage, may present this complicated aspect. As the case was not seen in the first stage, it is impossible to say whether it then presented evidence of that sudden and violent impression on the nervous system which characterizes an attack of acute cholera. Its subsequent course corresponded sufficiently well with the description of this variety, and especially with the modification of which has been proposed, p. 121.

The patient was a stranger to me and to the homœopathic practice. She lived in my vicinity, and probably endeavored to obtain the nearest physician, after failing to secure the attendance of her family physician, who was an allopathist, and who, by an office prescription, preceded me in the treatment of the case. The attack was about 10, P.M. I first saw the patient about 2, A.M., her physician not being able to visit her in the night. After the attack, she had taken, either by his advice or of her own accord, a dose consisting of ten drops of Camphor, mixed with a teaspoonful of Laudanum, what else, is not known. Collapse was already approaching, the pulse very feeble, and the cramps severe. For a more particular account of these, of the evacuations upwards and downwards, of the coldness and other symptoms, and of a remarkable phenomenon observed after death, the reader is referred to the Appendix, written by one who assisted in the treatment of the case, and who some years since had occasion to use it in an essay.

℞. Camph. $\frac{1}{10}$, a drop every five minutes. This with two doses of Veratrum ^{12}, and ^{30}, and two of Cuprum ^{30}, constituted the treatment for the first two hours after we were called. Then Secale ^{12} and Cuprum ^{30}. Afterwards, about five doses Camph. $\frac{1}{10}$, gt. j. as before.

CASE 23.—Monday, July 30th, 1849. A girl, aged 8 years, was well till four o'clock this morning; then diarrhœa commenced. Four brown stools of a gruelly consistence, in four and three quarter hours, at the end of which time she was first visited, and found in a state of collapse. There had not been more than a quart of the stools in all—i. e. one-half pint each. The body was almost universally cold, quite as cold as a corpse usually is several minutes after death, and covered with a cold and clammy perspiration. Face bluish, and hands bluish and wrinkled. Desire for ice. Voice reduced to a whisper.

℞. Camph. gt. j. every five minutes. After about four of these one-drop doses, she had a serous stool with a copious ricey sediment. But the whole was only about a gill and a half, i. e. six ounces.

There is no farther record of the treatment. The patient died about noon, about three hours from the time of the physician's first visit, and eight hours after the attack, no medical assistance was applied for until collapse had taken place.

Remarks.—The discharges were not such, either in quantity, consistence or color, as to justify us in considering this a case of Cholera, unless the other symptoms had been present. This, and the following case, in which the result was favorable, were under the treatment of my son, B. F. Joslin, Jr.; but as he was at that time an under-graduate, they were reported and numbered with mine. I saw them in consultation. Both cases were acute in the suddenness of the invasion, and the rapidity of their progress to collapse, and this one at least, without any adequate cause in the quantity of the evacuations. They were not even ricey or watery, until after full collapse had been established and the treatment commenced, and there was no evidence of any considerable amount of serous material that had been until then retained.

CASE 24.—A girl, aged 7½, was attacked about four and a half, P. M., Thursday, Aug. 16th, 1849. The disease commenced with diarrhœa and vomiting. Was seen before the collapse was complete. Then took one-drop doses of tincture of Camphor, afterwards some doses of Camphor [3], then was treated with Veratrum [30]. She was in collapse within two or three hours from the commencement of the first symptoms of disease. Pulseless. Voice nearly lost. Tongue, face and limbs cold. Cramps. Urine suppressed. In the evening she was put under Carbo-veg. [30] and Cuprum-metal. [30], alternately every half an hour.

Friday, the second day, in the morning.—After remaining in this state of collapse for twelve hours, entirely pulseless, reaction came on in the morning, under the continued use of the Carb.-v. [30] and Cupr. [30] given as above mentioned. The pulse and voice were restored, and the tongue and most of the skin acquired a temperature nearly normal. The same treatment was continued.

Saturday, the third day. A stool nearly normal, except as to consistence, which was that of mush—i. e. semi-fluid. Reaction about complete. Temperature normal. The recovery was oson complete.

Remarks.—This case, in respect to the rapidity with which the patient sank into collapse, was more acute than the preceding. The amount of evacuations was not definitely ascertained, but could not have been remarkable. As in the preceding case, my son was the attending physician, and I visited in consultation.

The locality in which this case occurred was extremely unfavorable, and the disease there remarkably malignant and fatal, especially under the old treatment. I learned from the father of the above child, who, though poor, was a respectable and intelligent American, that all the cases which had occurred in that filthy, blind alley or court-yard, and had been treated allopathically either there or at the hospitals, had died.* Being aware of the danger to which his family was exposed, he had represented the state of things (perhaps not fully) to the City Inspector, in May. At the commencement of the epidemic, there were four small adjoining houses, containing twenty-eight families, in this *cæcum* or blind hole, filled with the stench of three privies full of putrefying materials. Nine of the families had left in a panic when they saw so many of their friends and neighbors attacked, and that an attack there was the visitation of death.

* The number which had occurred previously to that time, the 16th, was said to be nine.

The privies remained completely full, and there were still on the 16th, nineteen families occupying the premises. In behalf of these poor people, I deemed it my duty on the occurrence of the above case, to represent the condition of the place to the President of the Board of Health, and to make a suggestion of a remedy. As this may be of use to others, at a time when to clean vaults may be as dangerous as to leave them full, I give from the letter, an extract relating to it.

"With the best means of preventing any deleterious gases and vapors from ascending from the vaults, the City Inspector is probably acquainted; but I take the liberty of suggesting a cheap preparation; which some gentlemen have used with great success. They take half a pailful of pulverized gypsum, half a pailful of pulverized charcoal, and one pound of copperas. When these have been intimately mixed, the powder is strewed over the sides and contents of the vault. It forms a crust over the latter, and keeps the air above, pure for a week. At the end of that time, the above quantity is to be again put into each vault. If the habitations of all the poor people of this city were thus protected by the Corporation, it would diminish the city expenses, and save many lives."

GASTRO-ENTERIC CHOLERA.

CASE 25.—Miss ——, aged about 27, was attacked Thursday, July 26th, 1849, at ten, P. M. At six o'clock next morning I was called from bed to visit her. The distance being a mile and a half, it was seven o'clock before she was prescribed for. She had had diarrhœa for a week, and checked it from time to time by brandy. At ten, P. M. of the 26th, after a tea of rusk, and rice pudding containing eggs, she had a large, loose alvine evacuation, which was followed by vomiting. The alvine evacuations and vomitings continued through the night and until the time of my visit and prescription. There had been eight or nine of each, that is the total number, upwards and downwards, was sixteen or eighteen. The stools were of a serous and ricey character—a watery liquid with a white ricey sediment. At seven, A.M., ℞. Veratrum ^{30}, in solution, every two hours, or after each evacuation, if they occur oftener. The patient was soon relieved, and was not again seen until three days afterwards, when, for some reason, not stated in the record, she took Phos. ^{30}, and six days after the attack, one Sulph. ^{2000}.

DYSENTERIC CHOLERA.

CASE 26.—On Wednesday, July 4th, 1849, I was called to visit a married gentleman, about 55 years of age. He had occasionally had slight cramps in the feet for about three weeks. On the 3d of July, at 4, P.M., diarrhœa commenced; stools brown and fœtid. Much pain in the bowels.

Second day, July 4th, nine, A. M. Has had two brownish stools. Tongue has a brownish yellow coat. I prescribed three Camph ^{3}, one every half hour, then Verat. ^{30} in solution, after each evacuation.

Four, P. M. Has had two stools since commencing the Veratrum; the last had the liquid rice-water appearance with white flocks, was without pain, but was preceded by cramps in the soles of both feet, and in the flexor muscles of the right thumb. Feet cold about the time of the evacuations, but reaction has come on: pulse now one hundred and eight. Tongue more moist and less coated.

Treatment.—Continue the Veratrum ^{30}, as before, *pro-re-nata.*

Ten, P. M. Stools scanty, and of bloody mucus with some whitish material. ℞. 2 Mercurius-viv. ^{12}.

Thursday, the third day, eight, A. M. Tenderness of the stomach and hypochondria. Has had several small evacuations in the night, with tenesmus and sense of pressing down. ℞. Sulph. ^{30}.

From this time the ricey and rice-water stools were intermingled with, and at length replaced by, others of bloody mucus in small quantities. The completion of the cure of the dysenteric portion of the case, required about eight or nine days longer, and was effected principally by Mercurius ^{30} and Sulphur ^{30}.

Remark.—It was not ascertained, that previously to the attack, there had been any thing unusual in the regimen or diet, except the eating of peas at dinner, on the day preceding the commencement of the diarrhœa.

CASE 27.—Wednesday, July 4th, 1849. Nine, A. M. A young married lady, was this morning attacked suddenly. First symptoms, liquid stools in large quantities, with pain in the abdomen. The first prescription was 3 Camph. ^{3}, one every half hour, then 1 Verat. ^{12}.

Eleven, A. M., second visit. The evacuations have been checked. The tongue has a thin yellow coat. ℞. Verat. ^{30} in solution, a dose after each evacuation.

Six, P. M., third visit. Since the last visit, only two evacuations. The stools small in quantity, watery and slimy, and the last one, at least, contained the characteristic ricey flocks.

℞. Veratrum ^{30}, to be continued, a dose after each evacuation, or once in two hours, if there is pain, even though the evacuations should occur at intervals longer than this.

Thursday, the second day, at noon. Stools of bloody mucus with some whitish portions. Pain and tenderness of the abdomen. ℞. Three doses of Aconitum ^{30} at intervals of two hours.

The patient was visited twice more on the same day, and received Sulphur ^{30} in solution.

Friday, the third day. The patient convalescent, and left under the action of the previously taken Sulphur, without repetition.

She recovered without any additional treatment, except one dose of Sulphur ^{1200} on the fourth day, two Nux-vom. ^{400} on the fifth, and one Nux-vom. ^{400} on the seventh, i. e. six days from the time of the attack. The convalescence from the dysenteric cholera commenced two days after the attack.

FEBRILE CHOLERA.

CASE 28.—A married lady, aged about 30, was attacked in the night, Friday, Aug. 10th, 1849, at three o'clock. Between three and eight, A. M., had five large, liquid stools, judged to be as much as a pint each; and the last one chiefly a perfectly serous liquid as to consistence, and of a yellowish color. I saw her at eight and a half, A. M., being called in some haste. She had taken five doses of Tinct. Camph. gt. j. each; and then, at intervals of one-half hour, two of Verat. ^{30}. She was lying on the sofa; rather pale, yet felt "feverish." Palms rather hot, both in sensation and to the touch. Slight pain in abdomen, considerable in the hips and limbs; some nausea. The tongue slightly red at tip; pulse about one hundred and ten; thirst considerable. Prescribed four doses Rhus-radicans, including the one administered. One to be given every two hours. Resort to Veratrum ^{30}, if there should be several large evacuations.

Five, P. M. Has had two more evacuations, thin, light-colored, and containing numerous white specks. Pain over the eyes, and in hips and small of back. Had taken Verat. ^{30}, once.

℞. Verat. ^{30}, each hour, until the evening visit. Improvement continued under Veratrum ^{30}, which was given occasionally next day, when she was recorded as convalescent, and on the 12th as recovered.

A case of Acute Choleroid occurred since the above was ready for press. On Monday, May 29th, 1854, in the morning, a lady had a stool of which the first part was normal, the last half-pint liquid. After dinner felt nausea, and a sensation of numbness instantly pervading the whole body, like an *electric shock*. The lips and fingers soon became *intensely blue*, and the latter strikingly *wrinkled*. The whole disease disappeared under *Camph.* ^{30} alone.

Cases 6, 15 and 16 also show the power of *attenuated Camphor*. If pellets of the 1st, 3d or 30th dilution supplant the tincture, we may avoid the *congestions*, which the latter sometimes occasions, also the *adulteration* of our medicines with its vapor.

CHAPTER X.

CHOLERA REPERTORY.

CONTAINING THE IMPORTANT SYMPTOMS, AND THE USUAL GROUPS, AND THE MEDICINES TYPOGRAPHICALLY DISTINGUISHED AS TO THEIR RELATIVE VALUE IN CHOLERA.*

EXPLANATION OF THE USE OF THE REPERTORY.

Believing that the success of Homœopathic treatment in Cholera, is such, that this book will be used by many physicians who have had but little, if any, experience in this kind of practice, as well as by many intelligent laymen, I deem it proper to explain the best mode of using the Repertory.

Select two important symptoms, of the case to be treated, and ascertain what remedies are common to both. If these are too numerous to be retained in the memory, write them down. Then compare this reduced list with the remedies as given in the Repertory for some other important symptom, and thus discover what remedies are common to the three. Then select a fourth, &c., and continue this process until there is only one remedy left. This will generally be the remedy for the case, especially if the symptoms selected are really the most important. The method of proceeding, thus far described, is the best for all homœopathic repertories, and if faithfully

* These symptoms and groups are frequently observed in cholera.

followed in reference to any disease, affords one of the best securities against that name-treating and *one*-symptom-treating practice, so general among domestic prescribers and hasty physicians.

In using this method and this Repertory in the treatment of Cholera, it will generally save labor to omit, at every step of the process, all those medicines which are not emphasized in at least one of the two lists. Such medicines will almost always be eliminated before the above process is completed. No medicine, which is printed either in small Roman letters or Italics, in *every* place in which it occurs in this Repertory, is, in the present state of our knowledge, known to have much power in the first three stages of non-inflammatory Cholera; and hence the use of such medicines, in Cholera, except by a very skilful practitioner, would be unsafe. If such should not all be removed by the process above described, the only safe course (at least for the beginner) would be, to commence anew, and repeat the above process with other important symptoms, combining them with each other and with some of those previously selected; and in general, the making of various combinations and in various orders, will give greater security in the selection of the remedy. If there are two remedies which apply to all the known symptoms of the case, the selection may be determined by the type in which their names are here printed. If the remedy is doubtful, and there is time for study, consult Jahr's Manual, especially the New.

One object in the construction of this Repertory has been to save part of the above labor, by occasionally combining the symptoms into such groups (of two or three) as the disease more frequently presents. For obtaining the remedies for these groups, the Materia Medica of Hahnemann, the Symptomen Codex and various Repertories have been consulted. The degree of emphasis has been determined by the clinical experience of the school in Cholera. I have, however, italicised some medicines which rank high for the symptom in general, but are not known to be useful in Cholera. The emphasis given to the medicines in this Repertory, has no reference to the 4th stage, nor to the inflammatory variety, except where it is so stated.

Medicines seldom used in any disease are omitted; also some for vomiting and diarrhœa, seldom used in Cholera, and found in Chapter XI.

The concomitant symptoms in any one section of this Repertory, are generally arranged in the same order as the sections themselves. Where symptoms, relating to different parts of the body, are in the *same* paragraph, those of the superior parts, are put first, and the more general symptoms last.

The paragraphs are arranged alphabetically; but where the same symptom, (as cramp) refers to different parts of the body, these parts are put in the natural typographical order, from above downwards.

MENTAL SYMPTOMS.

Anguish, anxiety or inquietude: Acon., ARS., bell., bry., CAMPH., CARB.-V., caus., cham., cic., coff., CUPR., dig., hyos., ign., ipec., kal., *lach.*, *laur.*, lyc., merc., natr., natr.-m., nitr.-ac., *nux*, petr., PHOS., *phos.-ac.*, puls., rhus, SEC., sep., *stram.*, sulph., tart., VERAT.

Apathy, or indifference: *Ars.*, bell., calc., cham., chin., *cic.*, hyos., *lach.*, lyc., *merc.*, *natr.-m.*, *phos.*, PHOS.-AC., sep., staph. *verat.*

Fear of Death, with internal Burnings, and tossing in the bed: ARS.

Taciturnity, or repugnance to conversation: ARS., bell., bry., calc., *cham.*, cic., coloc., cupr., ign., lach., merc., natr.-m., nux, *phos.-ac.*, puls., rheum, stann., staph., sulph., sulph.-ac., VERAT.

HEAD.

Confusion in the head: *Acon.*, *ars.*, *bell.*, *bry.*, calc., CAMPH., caus., chin., dig., merc., nux, op., *phos.-ac.*, puls., rheum, rhus, *sec.*, sep., sulph.-ac., tart., VERAT.

Heaviness, or pressure in the head: Acon., arn., *ars.*, bell., bry., calc., CAMPH., *carb.-v.*, cham., chin., *cic.*, dulc., ign., *ipec.*, *lach.*, *laur.*, lyc., merc., *natr.-m.*, nux, op., petr., PHOS., PHOS.-AC., puls., rheum., rhus, sep., sil., stann., sulph., *tart.*, VERAT.

Vertigo: Acon., ant., arn., *ars.*, *bell.*, bry., calc., CAMPH., *carb.-v.*, caus., *cic.*, *cupr.*, dig., fer., graph., hep., hyos., ign., *ipec.*, *kal.*, *lach.*, *laur.*, lyc., merc., nat., *natr.-m.*, nux, op., *petr.*, PHOS., PHOS.-AC., puls., rhus, SEC., sep., sil., stram., sulph., sulph.-ac., tart., thuj., VERAT.

Vertigo with *nausea* and *thirst:* VERAT.

Vertigo with *stupor:* Ars., *bell.*, bry., calc., caus., *kal.*, *laur.*, lyc., merc., *natr.-m.*, nux, *op.*, PHOS., *phos.-ac.*, puls., rhus, SEC., sil., spig., *stram.*, sulph., *tart.*, VERAT.

EYES.

Eyes sunk in the orbits; with livid semi-circles under them: ARS., calc., *camph.*, *cic.*, CUPR., kal., *laur.*, PHOS., PHOS.-AC., SEC., sulph., VERAT.

Eyes sunk in the orbits; with *hoarse* voice: ARS., calc., *camph.*, *cic.*, CUPR., kal., *laur.*, PHOS., *phos.-ac.*, SEC., sulph., VERAT.

Eyes Up-turned and Fixed: CAMPH., *cic.*, VERAT.

Pupils contracted: ARS., bell., *cham.*, CAMPH., *cicut.*, *nux*, *puls.*, SECAL., sep., VERAT.

FACE.

Bluish color of the face: Acon., ARS., bell., bry., CAMPH., cham., *cic.*, con., CUPR., dig., dros., hep., *hyos.*, ign., *ipec.*, lach., lyc., merc., *op.*, *phos*, puls., samb., spong., staph., stram., tart., VERAT.

Bluish and pale face: ARS., bell., bry., CAMPH., *cic.*, con., CUPR., dig., dros., hep., hyos., ign., *ipec.*, lach., lyc., merc., op., PHOS., puls., samb., spong., *stram.*, TART., VERAT.

Bluish color about the Eyes: ARS., calc., cham., *chin*, CUPR., fer., graph., hep., ign., *ipec.*, kal., lach., lyc., merc., natr., nux, *oleand.*, *phos.*, PHOS.-AC., *rhus*, sabin., SEC., sep., spig., staph., stram., sulph., VERAT.

Blueness of the lips: Ang.-spur., *ars.*, *camph.* caus., berb., chin.-sulph., *cupr.*, dig., lyc., *phos.*

Blueness of the lips, with corrugated and withered appearance of the skin: ARS., CAMPH., CUPR., *lyc.*, *phos.*

Blueness under Eyes: Sleeps with eyes open: Ipec., PHOS.-AC., *sulph.*, VERAT.

Blueness of the face and lips; Coldness of the lips: ARS., *cupr.*, VERAT.

Blueness of the face; vomiting after drinking; pulse slow; sweat clammy: VERAT.

Cold Perspiration on the face: *Carb.-v.*, rheum., nux, rhus, *verat.*

Cold perspiration on the forehead during the evacuation: VERAT.

Cold Perspiration on the Face and Limbs: CARB.-V.

Coldness of the *nose:* Arn., bell., plumb., *verat.*

Coldness of the nose and hands: Bell., VERAT.

Facies cholerica: ARS., *camph.*, *carb.-v.*, CUPR., ipec., *laur.*, *phos.*, phos.-ac., rhus, SEC., VERAT.

Face choleric; Voice hoarse: ARS., *camph.*, CARB.-V., CUPR., *laur.*, PHOS., *phos.-ac.*, rhus, *sec.* VERAT.

Spasm of the Jaw: Bell., *cham.*, CAMPH., *cicut.*, CUPR., *hydrocy.*, lach., *laur.*, op., rhus, SEC., VERAT.

TONGUE.

Coats on the Tongue.

Brown: Bell., CARB.-V., hyos., PHOS., rhus-rad., sabin., sulph.

Mucous: Bell., *cupr.*, dulc., lach., merc., PHOS.-AC. puls., sulph.

Viscid: PHOS.-AC.

White: Ant., arn., bell., bry., calc. *carb.-v.*, *cupr.*, dig., ign., *ipec.*, *merc.*, nitr., nux, petr., puls., sabin., *sec.*, sep., sulph.

Yellowish: Bell., bry., *carb.-v.*, cham., chin., coloc., IPEC., *nux*, plumb., puls., *rhus-rad.*, *verat.*

Coldness of the tongue: *Ars.*, bell., *camph.*, *laur.*, natr.-m., *sec.*, VERAT.

Coldness of the tongue and breath: ARS., CARB.-V., *camph.*, VERAT.

Coldness of the tongue, with *dryness* of it and of the mouth: ARS., bell., *camph.*, *laur.*, SEC., VERAT.

Coldness of the tongue, with *cold sweat* on the body: *Ars.*, CAMPH., *sec.*, VERAT.

The same symptoms in a more advanced state of *collapse:* ARS., camph., *carb.-v.*, CUPR., SEC., VERAT.

Redness of the tongue: *Ars.*, bell., bry., cham., hyos., lach., nux, rhus, stann., sulph., *verat.*

Redness of the tip of the tongue, in the febrile variety, or in the 4th stage: RHUS-RAD.

Tongue *Red*, and coated yellow: Bry., cham., *nux*, r.-rad., VERAT.

Tongue *Red;* Pulse Slow: Bell, rhus-rad. VERAT.

NAUSEA AND THIRST.

Nausea with *thirst:* Bell., PHOS., VERAT.

Nausea with *vertigo:* CAMPH., merc., *verat.*

Nausea with continued *pain* at the *pit* of the *stomach:* Acon., ARS., bell., CAMPH., *cham.*, CUPR., merc., *natr.-m.*, *nux*, PHOS., puls., rhus, *sulph.*, *tart.*, VERAT.

Nausea with *diarrhœa:* *Ars.*, ipec., *merc.*, PHOS.

Thirst, violent: Acon., ARS., bry., CAMPH., CARB.-V., cham., *cic.*, CUPR., *ipec.*, *laur.*, *merc.*, *natr.-m.*, nux, *phos*, *phos.-ac.*, SEC., *stram.*, VERAT.

Thirst, with *nausea:* PHOS., VERAT.

VOMITING.

Vomiting after a meal; blueness of the lips: ARS., *phos*

Vomiting after drinking; with blueness of the face: ARS., VERAT.

Vomiting after *drinking:* Arn., Ars., bry., *nux*, puls., Verat.

Vomiting frothy: VERAT.

Vomiting of a *watery* liquid, analogous to that of the stools, with pieces of *mucus:* Ars., bell., camph., Cupr., Jatroph., *sec.*, Ipec., stram., VERAT.

Vomiting with *pain* in the *stomach:* Ars., bry., *camph.*, Cupr., Ipec., *lach.*, nux, Phos., sulph., stram., *tart.*, VERAT.

Vomiting with *Colic:* *Ars.*, Cupr., *nux*, Phos., puls., stram., tart., VERAT.

Vomiting with *diarrhœa:* *Ars.*, *cupr.*, jat., Ipec., *phos.*, *sec.*, stram., tart., VERAT.

Vomiting with *Colic* and *Diarrhœa:* Ars., Cupr., Phos., stram., tart., VERAT.

Vomiting with *lassitude:* *Ars.*, *camph.*, Ipec., phos., VERAT.

PAINFUL SENSATIONS AT THE STOMACH AND PIT OF THE STOMACH.

Anxiety, *distension* and *pressure* at the pit of the stomach: Ars.

Burning in the stomach: ARS., bell., bry., *camph.*, canth., Carb.-v., cham., cic., jat., *laur.*, merc., nux, Phos., *phos.-ac.*, Sec., *verat.*

Burning in the pit of the stomach: Acon., Ars., bell., bry., *laur.*, merc., nux, Phos., *sec.*, Verat.

Burning Heat in the stomach or pit of stomach: ARS., Camph., Hydroc., Phos.

Burning sensation in the stomach and intestines, sometimes extending along the œsophagus to the mouth: ARS.

Cramp in the stomach: Bell., bry., *carb.-v.*, cham., CUPR., natr.-m., nux, PHOS., SEC., VERAT.

Pressure and Anxiety at the pit of the stomach: ARS., CAMPH., *cupr.*, IPEC, NUX-VOM., *verat.*

Continued *Pain* at the pit of the stomach with *nausea*: *Acon.*, ARS., *bell.*, CAMPH., *cham.*, CUPR., merc., *natr.-m.*, *nux*, PHOS., rhus, *sulph.*, *tart.*, VERAT.

Pain in the stomach, *with vomiting*: ARS., camph., CUPR., IPEC., PHOS., TART., VERAT.

Continued *Pain* in the *pit* of the *Stomach with Rumblings* in the intestines: Acon., *ars.*, bell., *camph.*, CARB.-V., CUPR., *jatroph.*, merc., natr.-m., *nux*, PHOS., PHOS.-AC., puls., *rhus*, SEC., *sulph.*, *tart.*, VERAT.

Pressive or *aching pain* at the *pit* of the *stomach with liquid stools*: *Ars.*, CAMPH., *cupr.*, PHOS., *sec.*, *tart.*, VERAT.

Pressive or *aching pain* at the *pit* of the *stomach*, *with cramps* or other *spasms* in the *extremities* or elsewhere: CAMPH., CUPR., *phos.*, *phos.-ac.*, natr.-m., *sec.*, *tart.*, VERAT.

Sensibility and *Swelling* of the pit of the stomach: Hep., lyc., *natr.-m.*, *sulph.*

Painful *sensibility* of the *pit* of the *stomach*, with *spasms* of the extremities: *Ars.*, CAMPH., CUPR., natr.-m., *phos.*, *phos.-ac.*, tart., VERAT.

ABDOMEN.

Pains in the *abdomen*, *with diarrhœa*: ARS., *cham.*, IPEC., *laur.*, *merc.*, *merc.-c.*, natr.-m., nux, *phos.*, rhus, stram., sulph., tart., VERAT.

Rumblings in the intestines: Acon., *ars.*, bell., *bry.*, *canth.*, Carb.-v., *cupr.*, *jatroph.*, laur., *lyc.*, merc., *natr.-m.*, *nux*, Phos., Phos.-ac., *plumb.*, *puls.*, rhus, *sec.*, stram., sulph., tart., Verat.

Rumblings in the intestines, with continued *pain* in the *pit* of the *Stomach*: Acon., *ars.*, bell., *camph.*, Carb.-v., Cupr., *jatroph.*, merc., natr.-m., *nux*, Phos., Phos.-ac., puls., *rhus*, Sec., sulph., *tart.*, VERAT.

Rumblings in the intestines, *with liquid stools*: *Ars.*, *jatroph.*, nux, *petr.*, PHOS., PHOS.-AC., puls., rhus, *sec.*, sulph., tart., VERAT.

Throbbings in the abdomen: Caps., ign., op., plumb., sang., *tart.*

DIARRHŒA.

Diarrhœa, with a *pasty tongue*, which *sticks* to the fingers: PHOS.-AC.

Diarrhœa with *nausea*: *Ars.*, ipec., *merc.*, Phos.

Diarrhœa with *vomitings*: *Ars.*, *cupr.*, *jat.*, Ipec., Phos., stram., tart., Verat.

Diarrhœa, with *vomiting* of the Food eaten, and of watery liquid: ARS., Cupr., Ipec., Phos., VERAT.

Diarrhœa, with aching or *pressure*, at or near the *pit* of the *Stomach*: Camph., cham., Cupr., merc., natr.-m., Phos., Phos.-ac., *sec.*, VERAT.

Diarrhœa, with pain in the Abdomen: Ars., *cham.*, *ipec.*, *laur.*, *merc.*, *merc.-c.*, natr.-m., *phos.*, stram., sulph., tart., VERAT.

Diarrhœa, occasioning great *Prostration* of strength: Ars., bry., *chin.*, con., merc., Phos., rheum, Secal., sep., *sulph.*

Diarrhœa occasioning great *prostration* of strength, in Aged persons: Con., SECAL.

Stools brown: Ars., CAMPH., merc.-c., sulph., *tart.*, VERAT.

Stools *greenish:* ARS., bell., canth., *cham.*, ipec., *laur.*, *merc.*, nux, PHOS., PHOS.-AC., sulph., VERAT.

Stools *grey*, or slightly whitish: Acon., *ars.*, bell., carb.-v., cham., lach., merc., PHOS., PHOS.-AC., puls., rhus, sulph., *verat.*

Stools *liquid:* Arn., *ars.*, *carb.-v.*, chin., *cic.*, *jat.*, lach., *meph.*, PHOS., PHOS.-AC., SEC., VERAT.

Stools *liquid* and *whitish: Ars.*, *camph.*, cupr., jat., PHOS., PHOS.-AC., *sec.*, VERAT.

Liquid and *whitish* stools, with *white* coat of *tongue: Cupr.*, PHOS., SEC.

Liquid stools, with continued *pain* at the *pit* of the *stomach: Ars.*, CAMPH., chin., *cupr.*, PHOS., VERAT.

Liquid stools, with *rumblings in the intestines: Ars.*, *jat.*, nux, petr., PHOS., PHOS.-AC., puls., rhus, *sec.*, sulph., tart., VERAT.

Stools *liquid;* evacuation *painful*, (attended with colic): ARS., *carb.-v*; PHOS., spig., staph., VERAT.

Stools liquid; evacuation *painless:* ARS., carb.-v., chin., *cic.*, PHOS., PHOS.-AC., SEC., spig., VERAT.

Stools *mucous* and *watery:* Ars., bell., chin., *ipec.*, nux, PHOS., PHOS.-AC., puls., rhus, SEC., sulph.-ac., *tart.*, VERAT.

Rice-water stools, or stools like *whey* or water, with *whitish* or greyish *flocks* in it: *Ars.*, CAMPH, *cupr.*, *ipec.*, *jat.*, PHOS., PHOS.-AC., *secal.*, VERAT. If there is inflammation, consult also, Acon., bry., and rhus.

Rice-water stools, or *watery*, *greyish*, *whitish* and *flocculent* stools, with great *thirst*: Ars., *camph.*, *cupr.*, ipec., Phos., Phos.-ac., Verat. If in the *febrile* variety, or in the 4th stage: Acon., bry., or rhus.

Stools *whitish*: Acon., ars., *camph.*, bell., *cham.*, *chin.*, cupr., *ipec.*, jat., merc., nux, PHOS., PHOS.-AC., sec., sulph., *verat.*

Watery and *white flocky* stools, with *cramps* and *thirst*: Acon., *ars.*, bry., Campr., Cupr., ipec. *phos.*, *phos.-ac.*, rhus, Sec., VERAT.

Watery and *white-flocky* stools, with *clonic spasms*: (spasmodic movements) and *thirst*: Acon., Ars., bry., Camph., CUPR., ipec., *phos.*, *phos.-ac.*, Sec., Verat.

Whitish Flocks in *serous* stools, with *pulse* scarcely perceptible: Acon., Ars., bry., Camph., Phos.-ac., rhus, Sec., Verat.

Liquid stools, with *white* flocks and grains, having the consistence and color of *tallow*: PHOS.

Stools *yellowish*: Ars., *cham.*, ipec., *merc.*, Phos., Phos.-ac., puls., tart., *verat.*

Yellowish stools, especially in an early stage of the disease: Ars., cham., ipec., *merc.*, Phos., PHOS.-AC., tart., Verat.

URINE.

Retention of urine: Camph., Canth., lach., op., plumb., Verat.

Retention of Urine, with ineffectual *desire* to urinate; at the commencement of the stage of *reaction*: CANTH., *verat.*

Urine *scantily* secreted, or *suppressed :* Ars., *camph.*, CARB.-V , CUPR., ipec., SEC., stram., VERAT.

The *same symptom* in the consecutive *fever :* BELL., *carb.-v.*, RHUS, *stram.*

Secretion of urine *diminished ;* with *cramps* in the *calves* of the *legs :* ARS., calc.. CAMPH., cann., *carb.-v.*, coff., coloc., con., CUPR., *graph.*, *hyos.*, lach., lyc., merc., natr., *nux*, petr., rhus, *sec.*, sep., sil., sulph., VERAT.

VOICE.

Voice *hoarse :* ARS., bell., bry., calc., *camph.*, CARB.-V., caus., cham., chin., *cic.*, CUPR., dros., graph., hep., *laur.*, merc., *natr.-m.*, nux, PHOS., *phos.-ac.*, puls., rhus, *sec.*, spong., sulph., VERAT.

Voice *hoarse ; face choleric :* ARS., *camph.*, CARB.-V., CUPR., *laur.*, PHOS., *phos.-ac.*, rhus, SEC., VERAT.

Voice *lost*, (aphonia): Ant., bell., CARB.-V., caus., cham., chin., CUPR., dros., hep., kal., lach., *laur.*, merc., *natr.-m.*, nux, petr., PHOS., puls., sep., sil., spong., stann., sulph., VERAT.

CHEST.

Anguish in the chest : Acon., ARS., bell., bry., *camph.*, *carb.-v.*, cic., CUPR., hydrocyan., *ipec.*, *jatroph.*, *laur.*, *natr.-m.*, *phos.*, PHOS.-AC., *rhus*, stram., VERAT.

Breath cold : CARB.-V. And, according to some clinical observations, *ars.*, *camph.*, *verat.*

Constriction (spasmodic) *of the chest :* CAMPH., caus., CUPR., fer., IPEC., lach., nitr.-ac., *nux*, op., PHOS., phos.-ac., puls., spig., *stram.*, sulph., VERAT.

Cramps or tonic spasms in the chest: Ars., bell., CAMPH., caus., CIC., CUPR., fer., graph., hyos., IPEC., kal., *merc.*, nux, op., PHOS., *phos.-ac.*, puls., SEC., sep., *stram.*, sulph., VERAT.

Cramps in the muscles of the chest, with continual *vomitings*, and with the *eyes turned upwards:* CAMPH., CIC., VERAT.

Respiration laborious; cold and *blue skin:* ARS., CAMPH., CARB.-V., CUPR., ipec., *sec.*, VERAT.

SUPERIOR EXTREMITIES.

Cramps in the *upper arms: Phos.-ac.*, SEC.

Cramps in the *forearms: Laur.*, *phos.-ac.*, SEC.

Cramps in the *wrist: Phos-ac.*

Coldness of the *hands:* Acon., bell., *cham.*, *ipec.*, *natr.-m.*, nux, petr., *phos.*, sulph., *tart.*, VERAT.

Cramps in the *hands: Bell.*, calc., cann., coloc., graph., *laur.*, *phos-ac.*, SEC., stram.

Cramps in the *fingers:* Arn., *ars.*, *calc.*, *cann.*, coff., dros., fer., lyc., nux, *phos.*, *phos.-ac.*, SEC., *stann.* staph., sulph., VERAT.

Cramps in the fingers, with clamminess of the tongue and skin: PHOS.-AC.

Cramps in the fingers, with clammy perspiration: *Ars.*, fer., lyc., nux, *phos.*, *phos-ac.*, VERAT.

INFERIOR EXTREMITIES.

Coldness of the feet: Acon., bell., *calc.*, caus., *dig.*, *graph.*, *ipec.*, *kal.*, lach., lyc., merc., *natr.*, *natr.-m.*, *nitr.-ac.*, petr., PHOS., plat., plumb., *rhod.*, *rhus-rad.*, *sep.*, *sil.*, *sulph.*, *tart.*, VERAT.

Cramps in the *nates:* VERAT.

Cramps in the *hips:* *Coloc.*, *phos-ac.*

Cramps in the *thighs:* CAMPH., *cann.*, *hyos.* *ipec.*, merc., petr., *phos.-ac.*, rhus, sep., VERAT.

Cramps in the *hams:* *Calc.*, *cann.*, *phos.*

Cramps in the *legs:* *Carb.-v.*, coloc., CUPR., JAT., *phos.-ac.*

Cramps in the *calves of the legs:* *Ars.*, bry., calc., CAMPH., cann., *carb.-v.*, cham., coff., coloc., CUPR., graph., *hyos.*, JAT., lach., lyc., merc., natr., nitr.-ac., *nux*, petr., PHOS., *rhus*, *sec.*, sep., sil., *sol.-n.*, staph., *sulph.*, *tart.*, VERAT.

Cramps in the calves of the legs, with burning heat in the stomach, or pit of stomach: ARS., CAMPH., PHOS.

Cramps in the *calves* of the *legs*, with diminished secretion of *urine:* *Ars.*, calc., CAMPH., cann., *carb.-v.*, coff., coloc., CUPR., *graph.*, *hyos.*, lach., lyc., magn., merc., natr., *nux*, petr., rhus, *sec.*, sep., sil., staph., *sulph.*, VERAT.

Cramps in the *calves; coldness* of the *feet:* Calc., graph., lach., lyc., merc., natr., nitr., ac., petr., PHOS., *rhus-rad.*, sep., sil., *sulph.*, *tart.*, VERAT.

Cramps in the *feet:* CAMPH., caus., graph., lyc., natr., nux, *sec.*, stram., sulph.

Cramps in the feet, with burning in the stomach, or pit of stomach: CAMPH.

Cramps in the *soles* of the feet: Calc., *carb.-v.*, coff., fer., hep., petr., *phos.-ac.*, plumb., *sec.*, sil., staph., sulph.

Cramps in the *toes:* Calc., fer., hep., lyc., merc., nux, *phos.-ac.*, SEC., sulph.

SKIN.

Blueness of the skin: Acon., arn., ARS., *bell.*, bry.,

calc., *camph.*, CARB.-V., CUPR., *dig.*, *lach.*, merc., natr.-m., nux, *op.*, *phos.*, *phos.-ac.*, plumb., puls., rhus, SEC., sil., spong., thuj., VERAT.

Blueness of the skin in different parts, and withered appearance of it: ARS., bry., calc., CAMPH., CUPR., merc., nux, *phos.*, *phos.-ac.*, SECAL., *sil.*, spong., VERAT.

Coldness of the skin: Acon., ant., arn., *ars.*, *bell.*, bry., calc., CAMPH., cann., canth., CARB.-V., *caus.*, cham., chin., *cic.*, *cupr.*, dros., dulc., fer., graph., hell., hep., hyos., ign., IPEC., kal., lach., *laur.*, *lyc.*, *merc.*, *mez.*, natr., *natr.-m.*, nitr.-ac., *nux*, op., petr., PHOS., *phos.-ac.*, plumb., puls., *rhus*, sabad., sabin., *sec.*, sep., sil., spig., spong., stann., staph., *stram.*, *sulph.*, *tart.*, thuj., VERAT.

The medicines which correspond both to *coldness* and *blueness* (of the skin), respectively or collectively, are: Acon., arn., ARS., *bell.*, bry., calc., CAMPH., CARB.-V., CUPR., *lach.*, merc., natr.-m., nux, op., PHOS., PHOS.-AC., plumb., puls., rhus, SEC., sil., spong., thuj., VERAT.

Skin *cold* and *bluish*, and covered with *cold perspiration:* ARS., camph., *carb.-v.*, CUPR., ipec., SECAL., VERAT.

Coldness of the skin, with mental indifference or tranquillity: ARS., ipec., NATR.-M., VERAT.

Withered or *wrinkled* skin: *Ant.*, ARS., bry., colc., *camph.*, cham., *chin.*, CUPR., fer., graph., hell., hyos., iod., kal., *lyc.*, merc., mur.-ac., nux, *phos.*, PHOS.-AC., rheum., SEC., *sep.*, *sil.*, spig., spong., stram., sulph., VERAT.

The medicines which correspond, respectively or collectively, to *blueness*, *coldness*, and *shrivelled* state of the skin, are: ARS., bry., calc., CAMPH., CUPR., merc., nux, PHOS., PHOS.-AC., SEC., sil., spong., VERAT.

The medicines which, on the ground of clinical experience, have been more especially recommended for this combination of symptoms, in the stage of collapse in cholera, are: ARS., CAMPH., CARB.-V., CUPR., *hydrocy.*, jat., SEC., VERAT.

PERSPIRATION AND PULSE.

Perspiration, cold: Acon., ARS., bell., bry., calc., CAMPH., canth., CARB.-V., cham., chin., cin., coff., CUPR., dulc., hell., hep., hyos., ign., IPEC., lach., lyc., merc., natr., nitr.-ac., nux, op., petr., *phos.*, *phos.-ac.*, plumb., puls., rheum., rhus, sabad., SEC., sep., sil., spig., stram., sulph., thuj., *tart.*, VERAT.

Perspiration, viscid, clammy: ARS., *camph.*, daph., fer., hep., *jat.*, lach., lyc., merc., nux, *phos.*, *phos.-ac.*, plumb., *sec.*, VERAT.

Perspiration clammy, with slow pulse: CAMPH., merc., VERAT.

Perspiration clammy, with spasmodic movements of the jaw: CAMPH., merc., *nux*, *phos.*, plumb., SEC. VERAT.

Pulse feeble and *frequent: Ars.*, CARB.-V., *lach.*, nux, rhus-rad.

Pulse Feeble and *Slow,* in the 1*st stage:* CAMPH., cann., dig., LAUR., *merc.*, puls., *rhus.-rad.*, VERAT.

Pulse Feeble and *Slow,* in the 4*th stage; Camph.*, cann., dig., *laur.*, *merc.*, *puls.*, R.-RAD., VERAT.

Pulse *feeble* and *small:* ARS., CAMPH., chin., dig., LACH., *nux*, PHOS.-AC., puls., RHUS, VERAT.

Pulse scarcely perceptible, with *watery* and *white-flocky stools:* Acon., ARS., bry., CAMPH., PHOS.-AC., rhus, SEC., VERAT.

GENERAL AND MISCELLANEOUS SYMPTOMS.

Burning internally, and *tossing*, with *fear* of *death:* ARS.

Burnings in the *stomach* and *abdomen*, with *anguish* and *tossing:* ARS., CAMPH.

Cholera followed by *cerebral* and abdominal affections: BELL.

Collapse so *complete*, that no vomiting, diarrhœa, or spasms remain, though some or all of them have existed previously; ARS., camph., CARB.-V., CUPR., HYDROCY., *laur.*, verat.

Collapse, without previous or present vomiting, or diarrhœa: CAMPH., CARB.-V., *hydrocy.*, laur., VERAT.

Cramps or other *Spasms* at *night: Ars.*, *camph.*, calc., cin., CUPR., hyos., *ipec.*, kal., lyc., merc., op., SEC.

Cramps in the *stomach* and *extremities*, with *coldness of the body* in an early stage, with but little diarrhœa: CAMPH.

Spasms, *Clonic*, (convulsions): *Ars.*, *bell.*, bry., calc., CAMPH., canth., *carb.-v.*, caus., cham., *cic.*, con., CUPR., *hyos.*, ign., *ipec.*, cal., lyc., merc., *natr.-m.*, op., *phos.*, phos.-ac., plat., rhus, SEC., sep , sil., stann., STRAM., tart., sulph., VERAT.

Spasms, *severe* and *clonic*, with but little diarrhœa or vomiting: *Ars.*, CAMPH., CUPR., ipec., *sec.*, VERAT.

Spasms, *Tonic*, (Tetanus, Cramps, &c.): *Ars.*, *bell.*, caus., *cham.*, CIC., CUPR., ign., *ipec.*, lyc., merc., *petr.*, *phos.*, *plat.*, rhus, SEC., sep., *stram.*, sulph., VERAT.

Spasms, severe and *tonic*, with but little diarrhœa or vomiting: CAMPH., CUPR., ipec., SEC., VERAT.

Spasms or *Cramps*, in the *extremities* or elsewhere, with weight, pressive *pain* or *aching*, at the *pit* of the *stomach:* CAMPH., CUPR., natr.-m., *phos.*, *phos.-ac.*, *sec.*, *tart.*, VERAT.

Spasms of the extremities, with *painful sensibility* of the *pit* of the *stomach: Ars.*, CAMPH., CUPR., natr.-m., *phos.*, *phos.-ac.*, tart., VERAT.

Spasms return at night: *Cuprum*, SECALE.

Excessive and sudden *debility: Ars.*, carb.-v., CUPR., *ipec.*, lach., *laur.*, nux, PHOS., PHOS.-AC., *sec.*, VERAT.

The patient *worse after midnight*, or early in the *morning:* Acon., ARS., bell., canth., CARB.-V., CUPR., kal., *lach.*, merc., natr., *natr.-m.*, *nux*, *petr.*, PHOS., PHOS.-AC., RHUS, *sec.*, stram., sulph., *tart.*, VERAT.

The patient made *worse by movement:* Acon., ARS., BELL., *bry.*, CAMPH., canth., carb.-v., cic., CUPR., dig., hyos., IPEC., kal., lach., *laur.*, *merc.*, *natr.-m.*, *nux*, *petr.*, PHOS., PHOS.-AC., plumb., *rhus*, *rad.*, SEC., stram., sulph., *tart.*, VERAT.

CHAPTER XI.

GASTRIC AND INTESTINAL REPERTORY.*

AUXILIARY TO THE CHOLERA REPERTORY, AND ADAPTED ALSO TO VOMITING AND DIARRHŒA IN GENERAL, AND TO CHOLERA INFANTUM AND DYSENTERY.

EXPLANATION OF THE USE OF THE REPERTORY.

THE arrangement of the symptoms of each section, is in general alphabetical.

* Taken chiefly from Jahr's excellent Manual, with some modifications.

The mode of obtaining the remedy for a group, is the same in this, as in the Cholera Repertory. The medicines seldom required, are here omitted. The emphasis in Chapter XI., has no special reference to Cholera; but in the treatment of this disease, this chapter may be consulted, when any case presents symptoms contained in this, but not in the Cholera Repertory; and that Repertory may be used as auxiliary to this and in general practice; for the medicines there enumerated apply to the symptoms, in whatever disease they may occur.

The 30th, will in general be a suitable dilution for most medicines, in ordinary gastric and intestinal diseases, for which this Repertory (Chap. XI,) is more especially constructed.

VOMITING IN GENERAL.

Acon., ant., arn., *ars.*, bell., *bry.*, calc., camph., cann., canth., carb.-v., *cham.*, chin., cic., cin., coff., colch., coloc., *cupr.*, dros., dulc., *fer.*, graph., hep., hyos., ign., *ipec.*, lach., laur., lyc., merc., natr.-m., nitr.-ac.. *nux*, phos., plumb., *puls.*, sec., sep., *sil.*, stann., stram., *sulph.*, tart., *verat.*

CHARACTER OF THE VOMITING.

Vomiting: Acrid: Arg., ipec.

—— Bilious, bitter: *Acon.*, *ant.*, *ars.*, *bry.*, camph., *cann.*, *colch.*, *cupr.*, *dros.*, *grat.*, *ipec.*, lach., *merc.*, *nux.*, *phos.*, *puls.*, *sec.*, *sep.*, stann., stram., sulph., *verat.*

—— Bitterish-Sour: Grat., ipec., puls.

—— Blackish: *Ars.*, calc., chin., hell., laur., *nux*, phos., plumb., sec., sulph., *verat.*

—— of Blood: *Acon.*, arn., ars., bell., *bry.*, calc.,

camph., canth., *carb.-v.*, caus., chin., cupr., dros., *fer.*, hep., *hyos.*, *lach.*, lyc., *mez.*, *nux*, op., *phos.*, plumb., puls., sulph., *verat.*, zinc.

—— of Blood clotted: Arn., caus.

Vomiting of Blood; sour regurgitations: Ars., calc., *carb.-v.*, *lyc.*, *nux*, phos., plumb., puls., *sulph.*

Vomiting Brownish: Ars., bis.

Vomiting of what has been drank: Acon., ant., arn., *ars.*, *bry.*, cham., chin., dulc., *ipec.*, nux, puls., sec., sil., sulph., tart., verat.

—— of what has been eaten: Ant., *ars.*, bell., *bry.*, calc., chin., colch., coloc., cupr., dros., *fer.*, hyos., ign., *ipec.*, lach., laur., lyc., *natr.-m.*, *nux*, phos., plumb., *puls.*, sep., sil., stann., *sulph.*, *verat.*

—— of Excrement: Bell., bry., nux, *op.*, plumb.

—— Frothy: Æth., *verat.*

—— Gelatinous: *Ipec.*

—— Green: Acon., *ars.*, *cann.*, *ipec.*, lach., phos., *plumb.*, puls., *verat.*

—— Milky: Æth.

—— of Milk used: *Æth.*, samb.

—— of Mucus: *Acon.*, æth., *ars.*, *bell.*, *bor.*, bry., *cham.*, *chin.*, cupr., *dig.*, dros., *dulc.*, hyos., *ipec.*, lach., *merc.*, *nux*, phos., *puls.*, *sulph.*, *verat.*

—— of Bloody Mucus: Acon.. hep., hyos., lach., nitr.

—— of Green Mucus; *Acon.*, *ars.*, *ipec.*, lach., phos., *puls.*, *verat.*

—— Painful: *Asar.*, tart.

—— Periodical: Cupr., nux.

—— Salt: Magn., natr.-s.

Vomiting Sour: Ars., bell., bor., *calc.*, *caus.*, cham.,

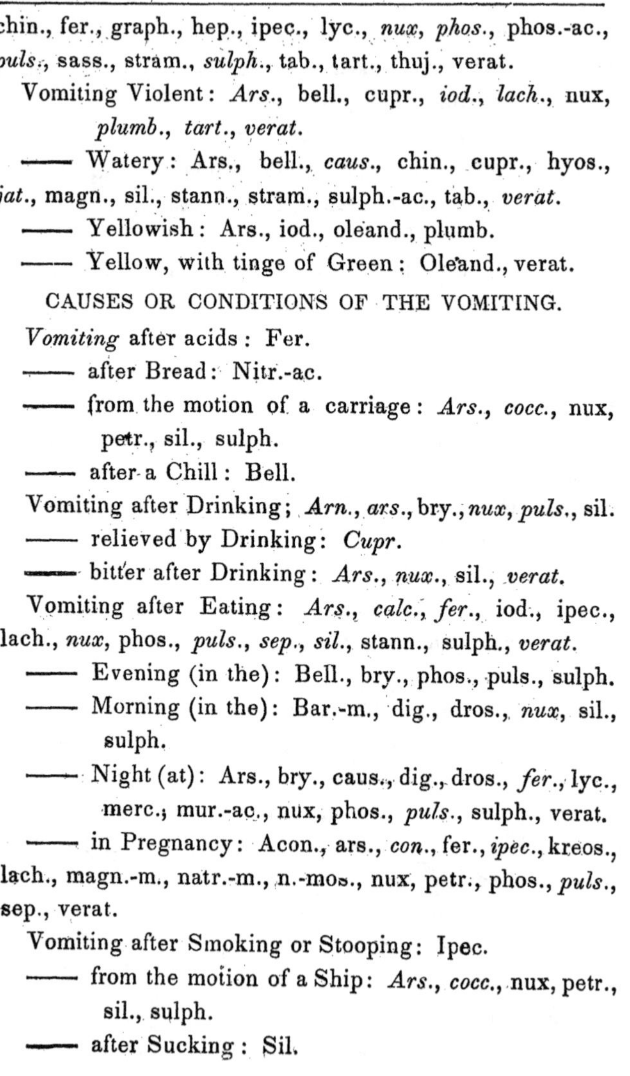

chin., fer., graph., hep., ipec., lyc., *nux*, *phos.*, phos.-ac., *puls.*, sass., stram., *sulph.*, tab., tart., thuj., verat.

Vomiting Violent: *Ars.*, bell., cupr., *iod.*, *lach.*, nux, *plumb.*, *tart.*, *verat.*

—— Watery: Ars., bell., *caus.*, chin., cupr., hyos., jat., magn., sil., stann., stram., sulph.-ac., tab., *verat.*

—— Yellowish: Ars., iod., oleand., plumb.

—— Yellow, with tinge of Green: Oleand., verat.

CAUSES OR CONDITIONS OF THE VOMITING.

Vomiting after acids: Fer.

—— after Bread: Nitr.-ac.

—— from the motion of a carriage: *Ars.*, *cocc.*, nux, petr., sil., sulph.

—— after a Chill: Bell.

Vomiting after Drinking; *Arn.*, *ars.*, bry., *nux*, *puls.*, sil.

—— relieved by Drinking: *Cupr.*

—— bitter after Drinking: *Ars.*, *nux.*, sil., *verat.*

Vomiting after Eating: *Ars.*, *calc.*, *fer.*, iod., ipec., lach., *nux*, phos., *puls.*, *sep.*, *sil.*, stann., sulph., *verat.*

—— Evening (in the): Bell., bry., phos., puls., sulph.

—— Morning (in the): Bar.-m., dig., dros., *nux*, sil., sulph.

—— Night (at): Ars., bry., caus., dig., dros., *fer.*, lyc., merc., mur.-ac., nux, phos., *puls.*, sulph., verat.

—— in Pregnancy: Acon., ars., *con.*, fer., *ipec.*, kreos., lach., magn.-m., natr.-m., n.-mos., nux, petr., phos., *puls.*, sep., verat.

Vomiting after Smoking or Stooping: Ipec.

—— from the motion of a Ship: *Ars.*, *cocc.*, nux, petr., sil., sulph.

—— after Sucking: Sil.

CONCOMITANTS OF THE VOMITING.

Vomiting with Anxiety: Ant., ars., nux.
—— offensive Breath: *Ipec.*
—— Choking: Hyos.
—— Colic: Ars., bry., nux, plumb., *puls.*, stram., tart., verat.
—— Convulsions: Ant., *cupr.*, hyos., merc.
—— Cries: Ars.
—— fear of Death: Ars.
—— Diarrhœa: Æth., ant., *ars.*, bell., coloc., *cupr.*, *jat.*, *ipec.*, lach., phos., rheum., stram., tart., *verat.*
—— pains in the Ears: Puls.
—— Eructations: Caus., mur.-ac.
—— Eyes convulsed: Cic.
—— Face, pale: *Puls.*, tart.
—— perspiration on the Face: Camph., sulph.
—— Feet, cold: Kreos., phos.
—— Feet, numb: Phos.
—— Hands, cold: Kreos., phos., verat.
—— Hands, hot: Verat.
—— Hands, numb: Phos.
—— Heat: *Ars.*, bell., ipec., verat.
—— Hiccough: Bry.
—— Legs, cramped: Nux.
—— desire to lie down: *Verat.*
—— Nausea: Nux, sulph., *verat.*
—— Pain in the back: Puls.
—— Pain in the stomach: Ars., *cupr.*, hyos., ipec., lach., *op.*, *phos.*, plumb., sulph., tart., verat.
—— Perspiration: *Ipec.*, sulph.
—— Perspiration, cold; Camph.

Vomiting, with rumbling: Puls.
—— Shivering: Bry., *phos.*, *puls.*, tart., sulph.
—— Shivering in the evening: Bry., *phos.*, sulph.
—— Shuddering: Verat.
—— Sight, obscure: Lach.
—— Sleepiness: *Tart.*
—— Taste, bitter: *Puls.*
—— Thirst: *Ipec.*
—— Throat, burning: Arg., puls.
—— Trembling: Nux, tart.
—— Vertigo: Hyos., natr.-s.
—— Weakness: *Ars.*, hyos., *ipec.*, phos., *verat.*

SENSATIONS (PAINS, &c.,) AT THE STOMACH AND PIT OF THE STOMACH.

Burning in the pit of the stomach: Acon., ant., ars., bell., bry., laur., merc., nux, phos., sec., sep., sil., sulph., verat.

—— In the stomach: *Ars.*, bell., *bry.*, camph., *canth.*, *caps.*, *carb.-v.*, cham., cic., graph., ign., *laur.*, *merc.* merc.-c., *nitr.*, *nux*, *phos.*, phos.-ac., *sabad.*, *sec.*, *sep.*, *sulph.*, verat.

Cold sensation in the Stomach or pit: *Ars.*, bell., ign., lach., laur., phos., phos.-ac., rhus, sulph.

Cramp: (See spasmodic pains.)

Sensation of *Emptiness* in the Stomach: Ant., ign., petr., sep., tart., verat.

Sensation of *Fulness* in the Stomach and pit: *Arn.*, *bar.-c.*, bell., carb.-v., cham., *grat.*, *hell.*, *kal.*, *lyc.*, nux, petr., *phos.*, *sulph.*

—— after a meal: Also, *chin.*, *merc.*, *puls.*, *sep.*, *sil.*

Pressure in the pit of the stomach: Acon., *arn.*, *ars.*

bell., camph., *cham.*, chin., coff., coloc., cupr., hep., ign., merc., *natr.-m.*, *nitr.*, *nux*, *phos.*, *phos.-ac.*, *prun.*, *puls.*, *ran.*, *ran.-sc.*, *rhod.*, *rhus*, *sep.*, *stann.*, *sulph.*, *tart.*, *verat.*

Pressure in the stomach: *Acon.*, *agar.*, *anac.*, *arn.*, *ars.*, *bar.-c.*, *bell.*, *bis.*, *bry.*, *calc.*, canth., *carb.-an.*, *carb.-v.*, *cham.*, *chin.*, *cic.*, coff., coloc., *fer.*, *graph.*, *grat.*, *hep.*, *iod.*, ipec., *lach.*, *laur.*, *led.*, *lyc.*, *merc.*, *mez.*, *mosch.*, *natr.*, *natr.-m.*, *nux*, *par.*, *petr.*, *phos.*, *plat.*, *plumb.*, puls., *rhod.*, rhus, *sabin.*, *sec.*, *sen.*, *sep.*, *sil.*, spig., *squill.*, *stann.*, stram., *sulph.*, *tart.*

Pain in the *Pit* of the Stomach, and in the chest, after a meal: *Bry.*

Pain in the *Stomach* and chest, after a meal: Chin., lach., phos.

Shootings in the pit of the Stomach: *Arn.*, bell., *bry.*, *kal.*, *nit-ac.*, phos., puls., rhus., sep., sulph., tart.

—— In the stomach: Bell., *bry.*, coff., ign., *kal.*, plat., sep., sulph.

Spasmodic pains in the stomach: *Ant.*, ars., bell., *bis.*, *bry.*, *calc.*, *carb.-a*, *carb.-v.*, *caus.*, *cham.*, *chin.*, *cocc.*, coff., *con.*, cupr., *fer.*, *graph.*, *hyos.*, *kal.*, *lach.*, *lyc.*, merc., *natr.-m.*, *nux*, phos., *puls.*, sec., *sep.*, *sulph.*, verat.

Swelling of the pit of the stomach: Acon., calc., hep., lyc., sulph.

Sensation of swelling there: Bry.

Tenderness of the stomach and region of the stomach: Am.-c., am.-m., ant., ars., bar.-c., bry., calc., camph., canth., carb.-v., caus., colch., coloc., hep., hyos., kreos., *lach.*, lyc., magn.-m., merc., natr, natr.-m., nux, ol.-an., phos., phos.-ac., puls., *rhus-rad.*, sil., spong., stann., sulph., sulph.-ac., tart., tereb., verat.

Tension in the Pit of the stomach: Acon., ant., cham., *nux.*

—— in the Stomach: Acon., bry., carb.-v., kal., merc., staph.

Throbbings in the region of the stomach: Acon., bell., kal., *puls.*, rhus., sep., sulph., tart., thuy.

DIARRHŒA IN GENERAL.

Acon., alum., am.-m., ant., arn., *ars.*, bell., bor., bry., *calc.*, carb.-v., *cham.*, *chin.*, cic., coff., coloc., con., cupr., dig., dros., dulc., fer., graph., hep., hyos., ign., ipec., *lach.*, laur., lyc., *merc.*, natr.-m., nitr.-ac., nux., petr., *phos.*, *phos-ac.*, *puls.*, rheum., *rhus.*, sep., sil., stram., *sulph.*, sulph.-ac., *verat.*

COLOR OF THE FÆCES.

Color, Black: *Ars.*, bry., calc., camph., *chin.*, ipec., merc., nux., op., phos., stram., sulph., sulph.-ac., verat.

—— Brownish: Ars., camph., dulc., magn., magn.-m., merc.-c., rheum., rhus-rad., sulph., verat.

—— Clay-like: Calc., hep.

—— Greyish: Merc., phos., phos.-ac., rheum.

—— Greenish: *Ars.*, *bell.*, *cham.*, coloc., dulc., hep., ipec., magn., magn.-m., *merc.*, merc.-c., nux., *phos.*, phos.-ac., *puls.*, rheum., sep., *sulph.*, sulph.-ac., *verat.*

—— Pale: Carb.-v., lyc.

—— Whitish: *Acon.*, ars., calc., caust., *cham.*, *chin.*, *colch.*, *cop.*, *dig.*, *hep.*, *ign.*, iod., nux., phos., phos.-ac., *puls.*, rhus, spig., spong., *sulph.*

—— White, like milk: Arn., *bell.*, dulc., merc., nux, rheum.

—— White, like flocks: Vide, *Cholera Repertory.*

—— White, in streaks: Rhus-tox.

—— Yellowish: *Ars.*, calc., *cham.*, chin., cocc., coloc., ign., ipec., merc., phos., plumb., puls., sulph., terb.

—— Yellow, in streaks: Rhus-tox.

ODOR OF THE FÆCES.

Odor: Corpse-like: Sil., Carb.-v.

—— Fœtid: Ars., calc., cham., coloc., lach., merc., merc.-c., nitr.-ac., nux, op., phos.-ac., plumb., rheum., sep., squill., sulph.-ac., tab.

—— Putrid: Ars., bry., carb.-v., cham., chin., coloc., graph., *merc.*, nitr.-ac., nux, sep., sulph., sulph.-ac.

—— Sour: Arn., calc., coloc., graph., magn., *merc.*, rheum., sep., sulph.

COMPOSITION AND CONSISTENCE OF THE FÆCES.

Fæces: acrid: Ars., cham., fer., lach., *merc.*, puls. sass., verat.

—— Bilious: Ars., dulc., ipec., *merc.*, merc.-c., puls.

—— Bloody: Arn., ars., caps., carb.-v., colch., coloc., dulc., *ipec.*, lach., *merc.*, merc.-c., *nitr.-ac.*, *nux.*

—— Coated with Blood: Con., magn.-m., nux, squill., thuy.

—— Burning: Ars., lach., *merc.*

—— Clay-like: Calc.

—— Corrosive: See *Acrid.*

—— not Digested: Arn., ars., bry., calc., cham., chin.,

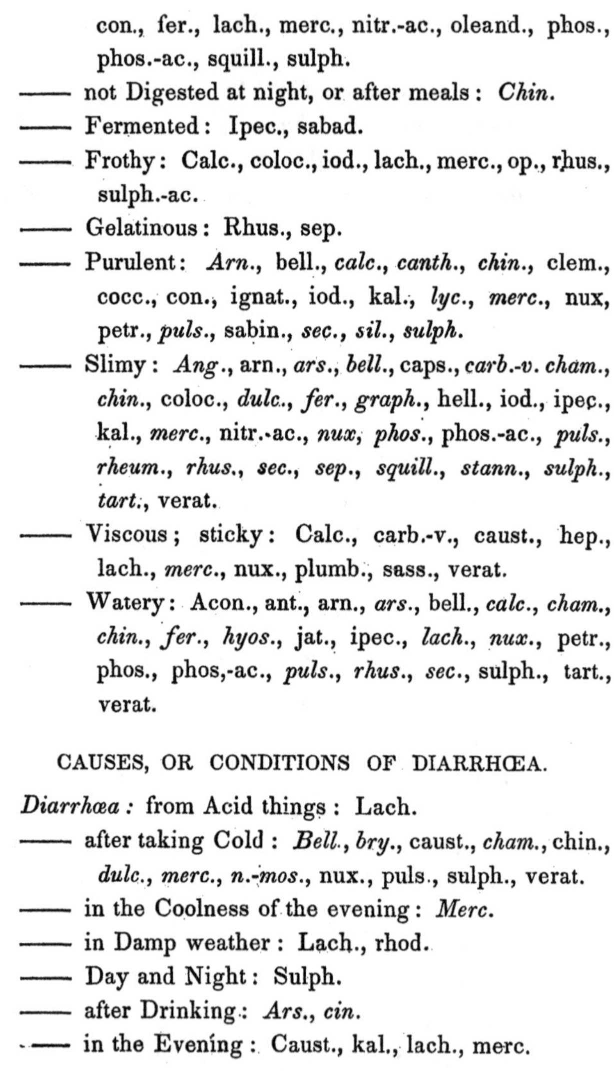

con., fer., lach., merc., nitr.-ac., oleand., phos., phos.-ac., squill., sulph.

—— not Digested at night, or after meals: *Chin.*

—— Fermented: Ipec., sabad.

—— Frothy: Calc., coloc., iod., lach., merc., op., rhus., sulph.-ac.

—— Gelatinous: Rhus., sep.

—— Purulent: *Arn.*, bell., *calc.*, *canth.*, *chin.*, clem., cocc., con., ignat., iod., kal., *lyc.*, *merc.*, nux, petr., *puls.*, sabin., *sec.*, *sil.*, *sulph.*

—— Slimy: *Ang.*, arn., *ars.*, *bell.*, caps., *carb.-v. cham.*, *chin.*, coloc., *dulc.*, *fer.*, *graph.*, hell., iod., ipec., kal., *merc.*, nitr.-ac., *nux*, *phos.*, phos.-ac., *puls.*, *rheum.*, *rhus.*, *sec.*, *sep.*, *squill.*, *stann.*, *sulph.*, *tart.*, verat.

—— Viscous; sticky: Calc., carb.-v., caust., hep., lach., *merc.*, nux., plumb., sass., verat.

—— Watery: Acon., ant., arn., *ars.*, bell., *calc.*, *cham.*, *chin.*, *fer.*, *hyos.*, jat., ipec., *lach.*, *nux.*, petr., phos., phos,-ac., *puls.*, *rhus.*, *sec.*, sulph., tart., verat.

CAUSES, OR CONDITIONS OF DIARRHŒA.

Diarrhœa: from Acid things: Lach.

—— after taking Cold: *Bell.*, *bry.*, caust., *cham.*, chin., *dulc.*, *merc.*, *n.-mos.*, nux., puls., sulph., verat.

—— in the Coolness of the evening: *Merc.*

—— in Damp weather: Lach., rhod.

—— Day and Night: Sulph.

—— after Drinking: *Ars.*, *cin.*

—— in the Evening: Caust., kal., lach., merc.

Diarrhœa, in Feeble persons: Chin., fer., rhus, phos.-ac., sec.
—— after Fruits: Chin., lach., rhod.
—— from Grief: Ign.
—— from Indigestion: Ant., coff., ipec., puls., nux.
—— after a Meal: Ars., chin., lach., verat.
—— after Milk: Bry., lyc., sep., sulph.
—— in the Morning: Bry.
—— at Night: *Ars.*, bry., *cham.*, *chin.*, dulc., lach., *merc.*, *mosch.*, *puls.*, *rhus.*, *sulph.*, verat.
—— of Old persons: Ant., bry., phos., sec.
—— of Pregnant females: Ant., dulc., hyos., lyc., petr., phos., sep., sulph.
—— of Scrofulous persons: Ars., bar.-c., *calc.*, chin., *dulc.*, *lyc.*, *sep.*, *sil.*, *sulph.*
—— when Sleeping: Arn., puls., rhus.
—— during Warm Weather: Lach.

CONCOMITANTS OF DIARRHŒA.

Diarrhœa with: Abdomen distended: Graph., sulph., verat.
—— Anguish: Ant., lach., **merc.**
—— excoriation of the Anus: Cham., merc., sass.
—— Colic, cutting: Acon., *agar.*, *ang.*, *ant.*, *ars.*, *asa.*, *bar.-c.*, *bry.*, *cann.*, *canth.*, *cham.*, *coloc.*, dulc., hep., *ipec.*, lach., *merc.*, *merc.-c.*, *mez.*, *nux.*, *petr.*, *puls.*, *rat.*, *rheum.*, *rhus.*, *stront.*, *sulph.*, *verat.*
—— alternately with Constipation: Bry., lach., nux., rhus.
—— with Cries and tears, in Children: Carb.-v., *cham.*, *ipec.*, rheum., sulph.
—— *Debility:* *Ars.*, *chin.*, *ipec.*, phos., sep , *verat.*

Diarrhœa, Eructations: Con., dulc., merc.
—— Heat: Merc.
—— pain in the Limbs: Am.-m., rhus.
—— pain in the Loins: Nux.
—— Nausea: Ars., bell., ip., lach., *merc.*
—— cold Perspiration on the face: Merc.
—— Shiverings: *merc.*, *puls.*, *sulph.*
—— pain in the Stomach: Bell., bry.
—— Tenesmus: Ars., ipec., lach., *merc.*, nux., rheum., rhus., sulph.
—— Thirst: Ars., dulc.
—— Vomitings: *Ars.*, bell., coloc., cupr., dulc., *ipec.*, lach., phos., rheum., stram., tart., *verat.*

THE MORE USUAL GROUPS OF DIARRHŒIC SYMPTOMS.*

Acrid and brown stools: Ars., verat.

Black and green stools: *Ars.*, ipec., merc., phos., sulph.-ac., *verat.*

Blackish stools after abuse of ipecac: Chin.

Bloody, mucous and fœtid stools: Lach., *merc.-c.*, sulph., sulph.-ac.

Brown and green stools: *Ars.*, dulc., magn., magn.-m., merc.-c., *sulph.*, verat.

---

* These, being nature's groupings, are of more practical value, than those which are formed merely from the Materia Medica, without reference to any observation of their actual occurrence in natural disease. The author, like most practitioners, has observed all of them in the latter, and most of them a great number of times. Those who practice accurately, often study to find the remedies adapted to groups: if they recorded and preserved the results of their calculations, the aggregate of those collected by different physicians would form a valuable repertory for general practice.

Brown and watery stools: *Ars.*, dulc., sulph., tart.

Brown stools, with nausea from movement: Ars.

Clay-colored and frothy stools in diarrhœa: Calc., rhus-rad.

Diarrhœa after fruit; with sighing respiration: Lach.

—— at night, with distension of the stomach and abdomen after meals: Bor., bry., caust., *cham.*, *chin.*, dulc., *kal.*, lach., *merc.*, *puls.*, *rhus-tox.*, *sulph.*

—— during dentition; white coat on the tongue; yellowish stools: Calc., ipec., *merc.*, *sulph.*

—— painless and at night: *Ars.*, bor., bry., canth., *cham.*, *chin.*, dulc., *merc.*, *puls.*, *rhus-tox.*, *sulph.*, verat.

—— with colic and at night: *Ars.*, bor., bry., cham., dulc., lach., *merc.*, puls., *rhus-tox.*, *sulph.*, verat.

—— with colic and tenderness of the abdomen: Acon., *canth.*, *cham.*, *merc.-c.*, *nux*, *puls.*, *rhus-rad.*, stram., *sulph.*, terb., *verat.*

—— with colic; stools fœtid: *Ars.*, bry., coloc., ipec., lach., *merc.*, nux, stram., *sulph.*

—— with colic; stools green: *Ars.*, bor., coloc., phos., puls., *verat.*

—— with white coat on the tongue, and yellow stools; Amb., calc., ign., ipec., *merc.*, oleand., petr., phos., puls., *sulph.*

—— with involuntary evacuations at night: *Ars.*, *bry.*, *chin.*, lach., *merc.*, puls., *rhus-tox.*, *sulph.*, verat.

—— with sweat on the face, nausea and stiffness of the neck, and pain in it when moving it: *Camph.*

Fœtid and green stools: *Ars.*, cham., coloc., lach., *merc.*, merc.-c., nux, sep., *sulph.*, sulph.-ac. tab.

Fœtid stools, in diarrhœa with colic: *Ars.*, bry., coloc., ipec., lach., *merc.*, nux, stram., *sulph.*

Frothy and involuntary stools, in diarrhœa: *Chin.*, merc., op., *rhus-tox.*, *sulph.*

Green and slimy stools: *Ars.*, *bell.*, bor., canth., cham., coloc., dulc., ipec., laur., *merc.*, *nux*, phos., puls., sep., stan., *sulph.*, sulph.-ac., tab.

Green, slimy and undigested stools: *Ars.*, bor., cham., nitr.-ac., *phos.*, *phos.-ac.*, rheum, *sulph.*, sulph-ac.

Green, sour and undigested stools: *Merc.*, *sulph.*

Watery stools, in diarrhœa with colic: *Ars.*, *cham.*, dulc., *lach.*, *nux*, puls., *rhus-tox.*, *sulph.*,

Watery stools with brown coat on the tongue, and vomiting at night: Bell., *phos.*, sulph.

CHOLERA INFANTUM, DIARRHŒA OR CHOLERA MORBUS OF INFANTS,*

Cholera Infantum in general: Acon., ars., bell., bry., calc., cham., dulc., hep., ipec., *merc.*, nux, puls., sep., *sulph.*, verat.

Cholera Infantum, with:

—— Abdomen distended: *Ars.*, *bell.*, bry., cham., *merc.*, nux, *puls.*, *sep.*, *sulph.*

—— distended, and pained during the evacuations: *Ars.*, bry., cham., *merc.*, *nux*, *sep.*, *sulph.*

Cholera Infantum, with Cerebral disease: *Bell.*

---

* The disease called Cholera Infantum, by American physicians, prevails during the hot season in the Middle States, and is often fata in cities.

Cholera Infantum, with Fever, thirst, hot and dry skin, pulse hard, and frequent: *Acon.**

—— with Stools green: *Ars.*, *bell.*, cham., dulc., ipec., *merc.*, nux, puls., sep., *sulph.*, *verat.*

—— with Stools yellow and slimy: Ars., *cham.*, ipec., *merc.*, puls., *sulph.*

—— with Vomiting diarrhœa and Slimy Stools: *Ars.*, bell., *ipec.*, rheum, *verat.*

It is unnecessary to dwell longer on Cholera Infantum in particular, inasmuch as the other parts of this Repertory afford a sufficient guide for the treatment of this disease; especially if the remedies for each symptom of the case be compared with the list given (at the head of this section,) as the remedies for Cholera Infantum in general. It is not, however, necessary to be confined to them, if the whole group of symptoms indicates some other remedy. Symptomatology, here as elsewhere, is the grand basis of treatment.

DYSENTERY.

Dysentery in general: *Acon.*, *ars.*, bell., *bry.*, canth., caps., *carb.-v.*, *cham.*, *chin.*, colch., *coloc.*, dulc., *ipec.*, *merc.* *merc.-c.*, nitr.-ac., *nux*, phos., *puls.*, *rhus*, sulph., verat.

Dysentery with dryness of the Lips: *Acon.*, bell., *bry.*, *chin.*, lach., *merc.*, *nux*, *rhus*, *sulph.*

—— with tenderness of Stomach and Abdomen: *Nux*, *puls.*, *sulph.*

* At the commencement of the treatment, Aconite is generally advisable.

10*

Dysentery, with tenderness of Abdomen: *Acon.*, *bell.*, *cham.*, *merc.*, *nux*, *puls.*, *sulph.*

—— with Stools of Bloody mucus, sometimes Green: *Merc.*, *merc.-c.*, *nux*, *puls.*, *sulph.*

—— with Burning in the Abdomen and Soles: *Merc.*

—— with Bloody mucous Stools and Tenesmus: Lach. *merc.*, *merc.-c.*, *nux*, *rhus.*, *sulph.*

For other symptoms and groups in any particular case of dysentery, see other sections of this Repertory, and compare the medicines, under each symptom of the case, with those for dysentery in general.

APPENDIX I.

AN ESSAY ON EPIDEMIC CHOLERA,

BY B. F. JOSLIN, JR., M.D.

PRESENTED TO THE UNIVERSITY OF THE CITY OF NEW-YORK, FOR THE DEGREE OF DOCTOR OF MEDICINE.—SESSION 1851–2.

THE early history of the Cholera is involved in some obscurity; for while some contend that it has existed in this country and in Europe only during a comparatively recent period, others believe firmly, that the epidemics with which we have been visited were only a more general prevalence of the Cholera Morbus, which is always more or less prevalent during the warmer months. In the descriptions of Cholera Morbus contained in the older books, the evacuations both from the stomach and bowels, are described as consisting "chiefly of bile." Any person who has seen the epidemic cholera, knows that in it the evacuations are characterized by an entire absence of this fluid; that though in rare cases, the dejections may be slightly tinged with bile, still in no case which they would consider as epidemic Cholera, are the matters ejected from the body decidedly bilious. A comparison of the symptoms enumerated as belonging to Cholera morbus, and those of epidemic or malignant Cholera, will I think, be sufficient to convince any one, that those diseases, though resembling each other in some particulars, are nevertheless not identical. The testimony of medical men who had had long experience, and who witnessed the first epidemic of Cholera, proves that the disease was one which they had not previously been accustomed to meet in practice. Watson says, (Prac. of Med. p. 407,) "the late Dr. Babington told me that it was quite new to him. He had for a very long period been in extensive practice in those parts of the metropolis and its vicinity where the epidemic Cholera raged most: and when it first came among us, he had the curiosity to ask every medical man whom he met, whether he had seen any case of the Cholera, and if the answer was "*Yes,*" he went on to inquire, whether before that year the person had ever met with the same complaint: and the reply was always, without a single exception "*No.*" Dr. Ackerly, who was physician to one of the Cholera hospitals in New-York, during the epidemic of 1832, says in his report, that "nothing like the late epidemic and malignant Cholera has occurred to my notice in twenty-four years practice."

Among those who believe epidemic cholera to be a disease essentially different from Cholera morbus, it has been a question whether it first originated in

India in 1817, or had been endemic there for a much longer period. That the disease which we know by the several designations of *Epidemic*, *Malignant*, or *Asiatic Cholera*, was known in India previous to the commencement there of the epidemic which traversed a great portion of the globe from 1817 to 1833 or 34, is probable from the evidence of resident surgeons and early writers.

As early as 1629, BONTIUS, a Dutch physician, wrote at Batavia, an account of what he calls "*Cholera Morbus*;" but from his description it appears to have more nearly resembled epidemic cholera. He says "this disease is attended with a weak pulse, difficult respiration, and coldness of the extreme parts; to which are joined great internal heat, insatiable thirst, perpetual watching, and restless and incessant tossing of the body. If together with these symptoms, a cold and fœtid sweat should break forth, it is certain that death is at hand." In his description of Cholera Morbus he says nothing of the spasms of the extremities, but he speaks of a person who died of this disease, as having died in convulsions. He also witnessed a disease that he calls "Spasm," which there is reason to think was nothing but the spasmodic variety of Cholera.

Dr. PAISLEY, writing at Madras, in 1774, speaks of "Cholera Morbus" as being "often epidemic," and accompanied with "*sudden prostration of strength, and spasms over the whole surface of the body*." He attributes the disease to the effects of "highly putrid bile;" but his description contains no information in regard to the appearance of the evacuations: his opinion as to the cause of the disease appears to be merely hypothetical. SONNERAT, who travelled in India, between the years 1774 and 1781, speaks of several epidemics of disease, the symptoms of which, as he relates them, very nearly resemble the Cholera as it has appeared in this country. He says, "the symptoms of this disorder were a watery flux, accompanied with vomiting and extreme faintness, a burning thirst, an oppression of the breast, and *suppression of urine.* Sometimes the diseased felt violent colicky pains; often lost his speech and recollection, or became deaf; *the pulse was small.*" Another epidemic, occurring two years after, "first showed itself by a watery flux, which came in an instant; and sometimes cut the diseased off in less than four and twenty hours. Those who were attacked had thirty evacuations in five or six hours; which reduced them to such a state of weakness that they could neither speak nor move. *They were often without pulse*; *the hands and ears were cold; the face lengthened; the sinking of the cavity of the socket of the eye was the sign of death;* they felt neither pains in the stomach, colics, nor gripings. The greatest pain was a *burning thirst.*" An English surgeon, Mr. CURTIS, in India, in 1782, described a disease which occurred in the national vessel to which he was attached. He enumerates most of the more striking phenomena.

of the cholera as being present in the disease he witnessed; as, general tonic spasms, the evacuations consisting of "nothing but a *thin watery matter*, or mucus;" coldness of the extremities, and subsequently of the *whole body*; the pulse "*sometimes sunk so much as not to be felt at the wrist, in two or three hours after the spasms came on;*" "in many, the stomach became so irritable that nothing could be got to rest upon it; but every thing that was drank was spouted out immediately; *without straining or retching*.

His account of the appearance of the hands in extreme collapse is characteristic. "The hands now begin to put on a striking and peculiar appearance. *The nails of the fingers became livid, and bent inwards; the skin of the palms became white, bleached, and wrinkled up into folds, as if long soaked in cold water;* the effect, no doubt, of the profuse *cold sweat*, which is one of the most pernicious and fatal symptoms of the disease."

He also speaks of patients retaining possession of their faculties "to the last moment of their life, even when the whole body had become perfectly cold, and all pulsation of the heart had ceased for a long time to be distinguishable." This disease can be shown to have been present in some part of India, during the period which elapsed between the last mentioned date and the year 1817, when it seems to have attracted more general attention than it had done at any previous time. From the above extracts we may conclude, that a disease similar to that which has visited us during the past twenty years, has been prevalent in various parts of India as an epidemic, at intervals during two centuries; and it is not unlikely for a longer period, though anterior to this we have no records.

In August, 1817, the Cholera appeared almost simultaneously in Calcutta and Jessore, in Hindostan, places about sixty miles apart. It is somewhat difficult to determine the exact point at which this epidemic took its start; but it is certain that within three months after its appearance in the above places, scarcely a spot existed within several thousand miles, in which it had not committed its ravages. In some localities the mass of the population was said to have been sensibly diminished. It is not my design to detail the routes pursued by this fearful scourge; suffice it to say, that its general course was westerly, though marked by many deviations.

Whether Cholera is or is not contagious, it very certainly has some other means than contagion of propagating itself; and its history has shown that neither non-intercourse nor rigid quarantine regulations were sufficient to stop its progress. I do not intend to enter fully into the discussion of the contagiousness of this disease, but will however relate the particulars of one instance, which illustrates my own view of this subject. On the second of December, 1848, the ship New-York, arrived at the quarantine, Staten Island. According to the report of

Dr. WHITING, health officer, this vessel had started from Havre with 345 passengers. About a week previously to arrival here, when off the coast of Nova Scotia, a number of cases of disease resembling Asiatic Cholera occurred, which terminated very suddenly. Out of seventeen cases, seven died. Subsequently to these persons having been taken to the hospital, there occurred in the latter place seventy-nine cases, out of whom forty-five died, making in all ninety-six cases and fifty-two deaths. Several of these cases were persons not having been passengers of the New-York. Among the latter was one of the nurses of the Institution. This is perhaps as fair an instance as could have been selected for an illustration of the peculiar habitudes of this disease. Here were a number of persons completely isolated, as a body, from the influence of contagion, and at a distance from any point at which the Cholera was then prevailing: it would be difficult to suppose any but an atmospheric origin in this instance. But further; the ship arriving at quarantine, where no cases of this disease had previously occurred, the disease still continues, and even attacks some who had never been in the infected ship: From whence did these last receive the infection? This last circumstance would seem to indicate that the Cholera was contagious, in a slight degree. From the above facts I deduce the following conclusions: 1st, that Cholera is propagated by means other than contagion; 2d, that under circumstances favorable for its development, the presence of cases in the immediate neigh borhood acts as an exciting cause. It is also worthy of being noted in this connection, that at least three persons died of Cholera in the City between the sixth and the twentieth of the same month, the first of whom had previously been discharged as cured from the quarantine hospital.

We may assume that Cholera is produced by a definite poison, without aknowledging the truth of any of the various hypotheses which have been brought forward respecting its absolute nature. This poison we know only by its effects; what it is, whether ponderable or imponderable, we know not: our only knowledge is derived from the effects which it produces upon the human system. Whether we suppose it to be, like variola, generated in the course of the disease and propagated by contagion, or produced by a generally diffused miasm, we may still consider it to be the effect of a *specific poison*. Acting under more or less favorable circumstances, we see this poison producing proportionate results: for though we might suppose the existence of this poison at all times, still without the coöperation of certain predisposing causes, its effect would not be general. That much of this specific poison does at all times exist in those localities which have been visited of late years by the disease, to me appears improbable; for as we have seen that there is no proof of its having often shown itself by the production of its effect, it must have remained latent under a multitude of circumstances which during the presence of an epidemic of Cholera seem to act strongly as predisposing causes. This remark is applicable to the periods intervening between the occurrence of the several epidemics, as well as to times previous to the first and subsequent to the last.

The *predisposing causes* may be comprised under the *meteorological* influences, the influence of *locality*, of *age*, of *individual habits*, and manner of living.

Meteorological variations have in numerous instances preceded the appearance of Cholera. Those conditions of the atmosphere which have appeared most to favor its development are, unusual conditions of heat and moisture, and alterations in its electrical condition. Thus its appearance would be preceded by long-continued storms of rain and wind, or by thunder storms. In other instances it has been known to succeed a long continuance of dry hot weather, especially if this state be succeeded by a sudden fall of rain.

The *localities* which have been most severely visited, have been low damp situations. Places situated near marches and upon the borders of rivers have been especially distinguished during the course of an epidemic.

Persons at about the middle period of life are more liable to an attack of this disease than either children or the aged. Young children are not unfrequently, during an epidemic, attacked with symptoms of the first and second stages of Cholera; but in them it rarely terminates in collapse; it is more common in these cases for the disease to run into a chronic diarrhœa accompanied with vomiting, into, in fact, *Cholera infantum.*

The following are tables, compiled from reports of the physicians having charge of Cholera hospitals, during the epidemics of 1832 and 1849. I have been unable to comprise all the reports of either epidemic; as only those arranged according to a uniform plan would answer my purpose.

Of 590 patients admitted into the Park hospital, during the epidemic of 1832, there were

11	patients	between	the	ages	of	1	and	10 years,
49	"	"	"	"	"	10	"	20 "
178	"	"	"	"	"	20	"	30 "
174	"	"	"	"	"	30	"	40 "
91	"	"	"	"	"	40	"	50 "
53	"	"	"	"	"	50	"	60 "
28	"	"	"	"	"	60	"	70 "
6	"	"	"	"	"	70	"	90 "

Of 407 patients admitted into the Rivington-street hospital,

5	were	between	the	ages	of	1 month	and	1 year,
42	"	"	"	"	"	1 year	and	10 years,
41	"	"	"	"	"	10 "	"	20 "
116	"	"	"	"	"	20 "	"	30 "
102	"	"	"	"	"	30 "	"	40 "
66	"	"	"	"	"	40 "	"	50 "
21	"	"	"	"	"	50 "	"	60 "

2 were between the ages of 70 and 80 years,
1 " " " " " 80 " 90 "

Of 281 patients in Corlear's Hook hospital, there were 25 under 14 years of age,

9	between	14	and	20	years,
84	"	20	"	30	"
88	"	30	"	40	"
47	"	40	"	50	"
12	"	50	"	60	"
14	"	60	"	70	"

2 who were over 70 years of age.

From the above it will be perceived, that there is very little difference between the liability of persons to an attack of Cholera between 20 and 30 years and of those between 30 and 40 years. The foregoing are from the reports of the epidemic of 1832, It is interesting to observe how nearly the following, taken from the reports of 1849, resemble them.

Centre-street hospital received 483 cases :

53	under	20	years of age,				
279	between	20	and	40	years	of	age,
141	"	40	"	60	"	"	"
10	"	60	"	70	"	"	"

Thirteenth-street hospital received 275 patients, of whom 63 were under 20 years of age,

157	between	20	and	40	years,
48	"	40	"	60	"
7	"	60	"	80	"

The remarkable similarity in regard to the relative proportion of those attacked at certain ages in 1832 and 1849, is shown in the following synopsis of the preceding tables.

In 1832, 14 per cent. of those attacked were under 20 years of age,

58 per cent. were between 20 and 40 years,
22 " " " 40 " 60 "
4 " were over 60 years of age.

In 1849, 15 per cent. were under 20 years,
60 " between 20 and 40 years,
21 " " 40 " 60 "
2 " were over 60 years.

Thus it will be perceived, that the greatest number attacked were of persons between the ages of 20 and 40 years. In proportion to the number of persons living at a certain age, probably a less number are attacked of those under 20 years, than during any other period of the same length. It would appear as if the aged were in some degree exempt from its influence; but if we take into consideration the small proportion of persons in a city over 60 years of age, it will be seen that their liability to Cholera is quite as great as that of those under 20. To illustrate the comparative *mortality* of certain ages I have prepared the following tables by combining the hospital reports of 1832 and 1849.

AGE.	NUMBER OF CASES.	CURED.	DIED.	PER CENT. OF DEATHS.
Under 10 years	58	31	27	46
Between 10 and 20 years .	122	79	43	35
" 20 " 40 "	788	367	421	53
" 40 " 60 "	194	72	122	63
Over 60 years	27	11	16	69

The *mortality* increases from *youth* to *old age*, as shown by the per-centage in this table.

The consideration of the influence of the habits and manner of living which predispose to this complaint, is important as guiding us to a knowledge of the true means of prevention. Not being wholly arrested in its progress by non-intercourse with affected localities, nor often held in check by quarantine regulations, it is evident that the security, either of individuals, or of masses of men, is only to be attained by removing from themselves, as far as possible, every cause which may be liable to act as a predisponent. Any thing which tends to diminish the general tone of the system, acts as a predisposing cause; irregularity of living, or dissipation of any kind, long watching with the sick, exposure to night air, and anxiety of mind, are all unfavorable. Of all occupations, that of a physician during the prevalence of an epidemic of Cholera, pre-eminently disposes to an attack; liable to be called upon at all hours of the day to visit the sick, not unfrequently in crowded and ill-ventilated apartments, compelled to undergo fatigue and loss of sleep, and to take his meals at irregular hours, it is not surprising that many of this profession are numbered among its victims. Nurses and those who attend upon the sick are of course exposed in some degree, not so much in consequence of the infectious character of the disease, as owing to the fact that such persons are liable to be deprived of proper rest and pure air. When several persons occupy one room not very well ventilated, as is too frequently the case in large cities, they are very much exposed during an epidemic, particularly if the situation be low and damp. I have remarked that the dissipated were frequent subjects. This is the case; but of all vices none predisposes in so great a degree as *intemperance:* this has been remarked by almost every writer upon Cholera. Of 1615 cases received into Cholera hospitals in the epidemic of 1832, 1023 were decidedly intemperate, a proportion of nearly two-thirds: of the remainder, 482 were intemperate: and of 110 cases, it was not known whether they were intemperate or not; it is probable that a proportion were. Both in the epidemic of 1832 and in that of 1849, the Cholera in New-York first appeared and was more fatal in the locality known as the "Five Points;" a fact which illustrates what has been previously said of its predisposing causes; this place possessing in itself all the elements best fitted for its reception, being low and damp, and the inhabitants filthy in the last degree. Among the *occasional* causes, we may enumerate the eating of indigestible food, exposure to great fatigue, and a depressed state of the mind.

For the purpose of description, we may divide Cholera into *three stages* or periods. The first stage I shall call *choleroid*, it may be also called the incipient stage. The second is the period of *full development*, and the third the stage of *collapse;* should the patient survive this stage, we will have the period of *reaction.* Either of these stages, *choleroid, full development*, or *collapse*, may occur without being preceded or succeeded by either of the others. This remark is more strictly true as applied to the first two periods; though numerous cases of collapse have occurred, without having been preceded by any precursory symptoms sufficient to excite apprehension either in physician or patient. The term *cholerine* is usually applied to the diarrhœa which prevails during the presence of an epidemic of Cholera, and which is properly the first stage of the disease. I have employed the term *choleroid* as designating the first stage, for the purpose of including a class of cases in which no diarrhœa exists. I shall define *choleroid* to be the occurrence of one or more of any of the symptoms of Cholera in an individual, only not sufficiently numerous or severe to justify us in considering it as a case of fully developed Cholera. The *diarrhœa* which prevails during an epidemic of this disease, does not differ in its character from the diarrhœa which prevails at other times when no Cholera exists. The evacuations may consist of ordinary fœcal matter, or they may be large and watery; they are scarcely attended with pain or uncomfortable sensation to the patient: this I consider to be the most distinctive character of the diarrhœa preceding Cholera. During the epidemic of 1849, instances occurred, in which persons would be affected with some very curious symptoms, apparently in consequence of the presence of the Cholera poison. These persons were affected by some among the more peculiar symptoms of Cholera. These cases are, I am satisfied, to be ranked with the diarrhœa, which we have been considering as effects of the Cholera poison, so modified by circumstances at not to produce its full effect. It was not unusual for persons to be troubled with slight spasms of the gastrocnemii, or of other voluntary muscles; these taking place in persons who were not ordinarily subject to them. But the more interesting cases, were those in which I observed symptoms of a more advanced period of the disease: thus a large number of persons had cold tongues, imparting a sensation to the touch like that of a frog's belly: and in one instance I observed the tongue to be not only cold, but of a bluish-black color, appearing as if it had been covered with ink. In my own person, I experienced some symptoms of a similar character to the above, which occurred several times during the continuance of the epidemic in New-York; and it may be as well to state, that I have never experienced them at any other time. The symptom most marked in my own case, was a blue color of the last phalynx of the fingers. The blue color was very decided, not unlike that of indigo. It was accompanied by some degree of corrugation, the appearance being precisely similar to that observed in collapse; it was generally attended with vertigo, which is not an unfrequent symptom in Cholera. These symptoms would last some minutes. I observed similar phenomena in other persons, only in less degree. The duration of the choleric stage may be only a few hours, or it may be several days. It is in this stage, that the disease has by all physicians been found most amenable to treatment, but owing to the salutary effect attributed to evacuations; under all possible circumstances, by the ignorant, this period is frequently altogether neglected, and the disease allowed to become fully developed before active means for relief are resorted to.

In the *fully developed stage*, the evacuations become large and colorless, or whitish and contain albuminous particles; they resemble water in which rice has been boiled, with particles of rice floating or settling in it. The patient ejects matters from the stomach of a similar character to those dejected. The matters vomited are ejected suddenly, generally without retching or nausea, and are frequently expelled with such force as to carry them to the distance of several yards. The evacuations frequently amount in quantity to several gallons, though the quantity does not have any relation to the severity of the attack.

I remember one case, which I saw in 1849, in which the patient was in collapse in three hours after the first symptoms were observed, and in which the patient died in about seven hours; the whole of the matters expelled from the stomach and bowels not exceeding three pints, and of a light brown color. Spasms of the voluntary muscles occur in this stage, which affect the abdominal muscles, the calves of the legs, the thighs, and frequently the muscles of the upper extremities and chest. Occasionally all the voluntary muscles will be affected. The pulse during this stage is generally less frequent than in health; it is not unusual to find it no more than 50 or 60 beats in a minute. The pulse does not vary much from its natural fulness until the disease is considerably advanced. The symptoms of this period may continue from one to twelve hours. When the disease is about to terminate favorably, the spasms disappear, the vomiting ceases, the dejections become tinged with bile, and perhaps acquire some consistence, or they stop entirely; in which event the patient may have no evacuations during the period of convalescence, which may be twenty-four or forty-eight hours. In some instances, the patients may have copious evacuations from the alimentary canal, without spasms; these are called the *Diarrhœic* cases. We have also the *Gastric* variety, when vomiting is the prominent symptom; also the *Spasmodic* cases, in which there may be no evacuations of any kind—only cramps. These designations are recognized by some authors, and are convenient in description; all agreeing in one particular, in their tendency to *collapse*, if not soon relieved by appropriate medical treatment. There is a class of cases which have been included in the designation *Cholera sicca—dry Cholera*: these are the instances in which we have the symptoms of *collapse*, without its having been preceded by any evacuation or other precursory symptom.

Collapse signifies an almost total suspension of the powers of organic life, not necessarily attended with loss of consciousness or impairment of the mental powers. It is the opposite condition to coma, in which all the functions of organic life are carried on, while the functions of animal life are totally suspended; we have a total suspension of the functions of the two principal secretory organs of the animal system, viz: the liver and the kidneys, two of the characteristic symptoms being an entire absence of bile in the evacuations, and a total suppression of urine, so that the patient will not pass the smallest quantity during the period of collapse. The other secretions are diminished, if not altogether suspended; thus though there may be the greatest suffering from spasms of the voluntary muscles, or from a sensation of internal heat, and from an insatiable thirst, the patient will not shed tears. There is an apparent exception to the absence of secretions, in the discharges from the alimentary canal; but even this is suspended in *extreme* collapse. The functions of respiration and circulation, though not entirely suspended, are nevertheless carried on in an extremely imperfect manner; the principal objects of these functions, viz: the oxygenation of the blood and the maintenance of a uniform temperature, being but partially accomplished; as is shown by the blue color of the surface, by the coldness of air expired from the lungs, and by the general coldness of the body. We must, however, consider that the mechanical portion of these functions is carried on more perfectly than the vital or chemical. These functions are not wholly subservient to the direction of the forces of organic life, but the function of respiration at least, is to a considerable extent under the direction of the will. While the functions of organic life are affected in so remarkable a degree, we have those of animal life remaining almost entire. The sentient faculties remain in many cases almost until respiration ceases; the patient can feel, see, hear, smell or taste, nearly to the last. The voice, being a function connected with respiration, is weak and sometimes scarcely audible, partly in consequence I presume of the diminished quantity of air taken into and expired from the lungs. The muscular system remains in great measure unimpaired, the patient being capable of performing many acts of voluntary motion.

In *complete collapse*, as seen in some cases of Asiatic Cholera, the features are pinched and the eyes appear sunken; the skin is of a bluish color, the whole surface being covered with a cold clammy sweat, imparting a sensation of *icey* coldness to the touch, the hands are corrugated, appearing as though they had been soaked in water for some time; hence this appearance has been called the "*washerwoman's hands:*" the voice is peculiar, so that it has been known as the "*Vox Cholerica;*" it becomes husky and faint; the breath is cold. The pulse is generally frequent, small and quick, sometimes intermittent and irregular. In many cases the pulse remains *imperceptible* for several hours, in other instances where it is not totally imperceptible, the sensation which it imparts to the touch may be compared to that which would be produced if the finger were placed upon one point of an exceedingly fine wire, tightly drawn between two fixed points, while something were drawn quickly across another point of the wire, producing minute vibrations. This I think illustrates the pulse of collapse, as nearly as possible.

The evacuations from the stomach and bowels become less and less frequent, as the symptoms of this stage appear, and in most cases cease entirely a few hours before death, in which in a majority of cases, collapse terminates. The spasms frequently continue after collapse has appeared, though they very generally cease a short time previous to death. The secretion of *urine*, which becomes diminished in the stage of *full development*, is entirely suppressed in *collapse*, and in post-mortem examinations the bladder is uniformly found empty. In this stage an insatiable *thirst* in many cases torments the patients, they taking drink frequently, but in small quantities; and while the external surface is cold to the touch, the patient complains of an *internal* burning. Among the characteristic symptoms of Cholera, is to be enumerated the stoical indifference which the patient manifests in regard to the final result of the disease. This apathy exists during the first stage, and increases with the progress of the malady.

The period of collapse lasts from two to twelve hours, and it may terminate in death, or be succeeded by *reaction*. Among the symptoms from which we may infer that reaction is about being established there are: a return of the natural warmth to the surface, and the pulse reappearing and becoming full and regular. A very important symptom is the return of the secretion of urine. The breath, which before was cold, becomes warm, and in fact all the symptoms which constitute collapse disappear.

It frequently happens that *reaction* does not stop until some degree of febrile action is set up; and here again we have another period of danger, arising from *excessive reaction*. In this period, the patient may have inflammation or congestion of any of the important organs of life, or again, it may be followed by continued fever. The most frequent inflammations are dysentery and inflammation of the brain.

In the foregoing description of Cholera, I have spoken of it as though it consisted of three clearly defined stages or periods: in a number of cases we find the disease running its course with as much regularity as the previous description would imply, but in a larger proportion of the cases which occur, this is not true, the symptoms described as belonging to the several periods being combined in every variety. Thus it can be said that no two cases are precisely similar.

The results of post-mortem examinations have thrown little light upon the nature of this disease; as but few of the lesions observed were constant. The only appearances which were constantly observed in autopsies of Cholera patients, were more or less of the rice-water and ricey matters in the alimentary canal, similar in appearance to that which had previously been ejected, and a thick black substance resembling in appearance tar, filling the veins, and the bladder was uniformly found empty and contracted.

Spasmodic movements of the limbs have been observed to take place after respiration had ceased. Instances of this kind are probably of not very frequent occurrence, as very little mention is made of them in works upon Cholera. My own attention was drawn to the fact by the following case which occurred in New-York on the 29th of May, 1849, about fifteen days after the first appearance of the epidemic in the city. The patient was the wife of a respectable mechanic, and was of perfectly temperate habits; age 40 years. She was attacked about ten, P. M., May 28th, having previously partaken of radishes for her supper that evening, which seemed to have been the occasional cause of her sickness. Symptoms: rice-water evacuations per anum; vomiting of a serous and slightly milky liquid, with pieces of radish, cramps in extremities, chiefly in calves and thighs. Tongue cold; urine suppressed; eyes upturned and fixed a part of the time; tongue covered with whitish coat, which afterwards became yellowish. The pulse was feeble, and became insensible two hours before death. Breath cold; feet, face and hands cold and moist, except palms, which retain some heat. Epigastrium swollen, painful and sensitive. Died about eleven and a half, A. M., 29th inst. After respiration had ceased half an hour, spasmodic movements occurred in her right arm; her fore-arm became flexed upon her arm; flexion of the fingers also took place. These motions were repeated a number of times, leading the friends to suppose that life was not extinct, and causing them to send for medical assistance. Another curious phenomenon, is the return of warmth to the surface, and its continuance for a considerable time after respiration has ceased. The temperature of the corpse, which previously to death was externally cold, becomes, in many cases after respiration has ceased, so warm as to impart to the touch a sensation of heat.

APPENDIX II.

HOMŒOPATHIC CHOLERA HOSPITAL.

As the Cholera has now reappeared in New-York and many other places, the republication of certain remarks, made on the above subject in 1849, is deemed seasonable and proper. As a majority of the medical profession retain the same prejudices, the friends of humanity and justice, here and elsewhere, will be again liable to encounter similar obstacles, in carrying out their plans for the relief of the poor, who are especially liable to become victims of this pestilence.

The great success of the homœopathic treatment in the cholera of 1849, by attenuated medicines, is now extensively known. When the epidemic had disappeared, the Board of Health of the city of New-York, through its Sanatary Committee, made a Report in which reasons were assigned for refusing to establish a homœopathic cholera hospital, for which a petition had been presented by hundreds of our respectable citizens.

Some of the reasons were assigned by the Sanatary Committee, others by their Medical Counsel, composed of several physicians of high rank. The parts referred to in the letter, are quoted in the words of the authors.

It will be seen that (to use the language of a distinguished writer) "though the Board, even while thus deciding, profess not to be competent to decide, they seem to consider themselves competent to sneer."

The Medical Counsel, in their report to the Sanatary Committee, say, that

"By intelligent and well-educated physicians generally, Homœopathy is looked upon as a species of empiricism. It is neither practised by them, nor countenanced by them. Concurring entirely with their professional brethren on this subject, the undersigned conceive that the public authorities of our city would not consult either their own dignity or the public good, by lending the sanction of their name or influence to Homœopathy or any other irregular mode of practice."

The Committee say, that

"In adopting this report, the Sanatary Committee do not wish to be considered as expressing any opinion either in favor or against what is commonly denominated Homœopathy. This they viewed as a subject entirely beyond their province."

After some other remarks, they end by saying,

"Taking this view of the subject, the committee felt it to be their duty to have nothing to do with medicine, except as they found it embodied in what is understood and known both by the public, as well as physicians, as the regular profession. While in this way they paid all suitable respect to so honorable a profession as that of medicine, the committee felt that they did no injustice to those who suppose themselves in advance of the age, and profess themselves gifted with superior knowledge and wisdom."

LETTER

To the Sanatary Committee of the Board of Health of the City of New-York:

GENTLEMEN :—In the report of your proceedings recently published, you assign reasons for not establishing a Homœopathic Cholera Hospital. Notwithstanding the equivocal compliment which you bestow on the homœopathists, as "those who suppose themselves in advance of the age, and profess themselves gifted with superior knowledge and wisdom," I shall assume that you intended "no injustice" toward either of the two great medical parties into which the community, as well as the regular profession, is divided.

The regular medical profession includes all those who have pursued the course of medical studies prescribed by the laws of the State, and complied with all the professional requirements of the medical colleges and medical societies which the State has established. The diplomas held by the homœopathic physicians of New-York, afford proof that they have passed these ordeals.

As such are the only tests of professional regularity recognised under this or any civilized government, I cannot presume that you "suppose" yourselves so far "in advance of the age, and profess" yourselves "gifted with" such "superior knowledge and wisdom" as to impose, intentionally, a new test not recognised by those laws from which you derive all your authority. How is it, then, that you refused to place one of the cholera hospitals under the care of regular homœopathic physicians, on the ground that "the committee felt it to be their duty to have nothing to do with medicine, except as they found it embodied in what is understood and known, both by the public as well as physicians, as the regular profession?" Is it possible that you were deceived by a mere name, which some physicians have assumed for themselves, and persuaded their friends to appropriate to them? Regularity, in its proper sense, is an excellent thing: so are catholicism and democracy: but I doubt whether you have all resolved to have nothing to do with religion, except as you find it embodied in the Catholic church, or with politics, except as you find it embodied in the democratic party.

You must mean, either that the homœopathic physicians constitute *no part* of the regular profession, or else that they constitute only a *minority*. The first position I have shown to be untenable. In considering the second, I assume that minorities have rights, on which no agents of government can properly trample. During a pestilence, the homœopathic citizens of New-York can justly claim, that a due proportion of what they have contributed to the funds of the city, be appropriated to the use of a homœopathic hospital. They have a right to dictate what provision shall be made for the treatment of the indigent and stranger of their own medical faith, so far as this can be conceded without infringing the rights of others. In regard to this last point, you were not requested to refrain from establishing as many allœopathic hospitals as you deemed expedient, nor to compel any patient to enter the homœopathic.

The statement of the main objection which your medical counsel urged against Homœopathy may be ambiguous; but it is susceptible of only two constructions: one is that "it is neither practised" "nor countenanced by" a *majority* of "intelligent and well-educated physicians." This proves no more than the equally notorious fact, that it is neither practised nor countenanced by the majority of stupid and uneducated physicians. Allœopathy has more great men and more small ones; for the same reason that white sheep have more wool than black ones.

The only other meaning of which the statement of the "counsel" is susceptible, is, that Homœopathy "is neither practised" "nor countenanced by" *any* intelligent and well-educated physicians. Is this the assertion of the medical counsel, a majority (i. e. two) of whose members are medical professors, who are annually recommending homœopathic medical students as qualified to receive the degree of doctor of medicine? From these and similar allœopathic professors, the homœopathic physicians now practising have received their credentials. When a professor affirms that his own certificate is false, to which of his statements shall we give credence? The case reminds us of the problem which exercised the sophists. When a man says, I lie, does he lie or does he speak the truth?

Neither the committee nor their counsel have attempted to refute the statistics by which the petition was sustained, nor to deny that Homoœopathy affords the best method of *curing the sick,* however much the "public authorities" might, by rejecting it, "consult their own dignity," and thus, indirectly, "the public good." Of their objections, I am not able to perceive any which are not substantially included in those which I have answered. If there is an appearance of mystification or muddiness in the whole train of their reasoning, I have too much respect for them to attribute it to anything else than the unavoidable difficulties attending the defence of a weak cause.

B. F. JOSLIN, M.D.

NEW-YORK, Nov. 17, 1849.

INDEX.

A.

B.

C.

F.

G.

H.

I.

Q.

R.

www.ingramcontent.com/pod-product-compliance
Lightning Source LLC
LaVergne TN
LVHW010253110826
845151LV00004B/1463

* 9 7 8 1 4 2 5 5 2 2 4 8 3 *